Brain Injury

Andrea Willemsen

my life after
Brain Injury

Published in dutch as a literary essay by Publishing house De Geus, the Netherlands: www.degeus.nl

ISBN 10 1503334880
ISBN 13 9781503334885

Original title: *Hersenkneuzing* by Andrea Willemsen.
Translated by Dennis Bailey
Advice on medical terminology: Dr N.I. Bohnen, University of Michigan
Translation grants: Dutch Ministry of Infrastructure and The RAI

The writer uses his pen to seize power, because the powerlessness is unbearable.

Connie Palmen, I.M.

Appearances can be deceiving. The appearance that the patient evokes in others and experiences himself. The appearance that he is his old self again and can be treated as such.

Prof.dr. R.A.C. Hoksbergen,
'Appearances are deceiving.
A patient with a fairly severe
brain contusion looks back'

for Willem Vrakking

Contents

Foreword 3
Introduction 5

Run Over 9
Sunday's Child 26
Written Off 34
Christmas 38
Neurological Patient 44
Next Time Stone-Dead Please 51
A Sheep On Its Back 57
Where Is My Head? 63
An Exercise In Pain 76
Balancing On The Beam 84
Letter To My Perpetrator 96
Recovery 104
Life With The Brakes On 117
In Training 123
A Life Alone? 136
The Great Silence 147
My Fellow Victim 152

Epilogue   164

Foreword

Research of brain injuries resulting from accidents only started some 25 years ago. For a long time the research and reports on what happens after this brain injury were focused mainly on severe, life-threatening situations. In recent years, however, science has looked more at the consequences of less severe injuries. This increased interest has shown that brain contusions that are less severe in medical terms, often have disastrous consequences for an individual's life. Gradually it also became clear that many of the consequences after an accident that were considered to be psychological or 'histrionics', were caused by actual injuries to certain parts of the brain, where, for example, emotions, memory functions or planning are located.

For those who have to live with these consequences it is important that they know how to do just that. How to 'cope'. For this reason it is important that individuals who are the victims of such accidents and are 'experience experts' can relate what they have experienced, how such an accident changed their lives and how they managed to cope.

Andrea Willemsen is one of these 'experience experts'. She has written a book. In doing so she not only provides a great service to other people with brain injuries, she also illustrates very clearly for professionals, physicians and paramedics how significantly a life can change. I am therefore extremely pleased that, despite her major handicap and after a lengthy writing process, she has been able to write a book like this one. And so I did not hesitate when she asked me to act as medical consultant for the Contusio Cerebri Fund (*Stichting Contusio Cerebri Fonds)* that she set up.

3

Through her book and the website www.hersenkneuzing.nl she has already provided concrete support to thousands of people in their search for information about the changes that can be caused by traumatic brain injury.

Prof. dr. J.M. Minderhoud,
Emeritus Professor of Neurology
(Academic Hospital Groningen, AZG)

Introduction

Deep skid marks have cut through my life since a carelessly speeding traffic offender on a moped knocked me off my bicycle one Sunday afternoon. At the time I was 43 years old, with an immense zest for life. I had a job as a scientific researcher and consultant, cared for my husband and two sons, was an enthusiastic hostess, played many sports and went to parties, concerts and museums. Since then, I have been obliged to back-pedal in all these areas. To this day, the brain contusion (contusio cerebri) I suffered in that accident still bars me from full enjoyment of virtually all my activities and opportunities. I lead the life of a very old woman, and half the time even that is too much for me.

So don't expect me to write a cool, objective account of my experiences. Obviously, I am sometimes emotional on the subject, and biased to the marrow. I burn with desire for justice. In our highly developed society, you bump into legal and medical regulations at every turn. But after my traffic accident the authorities who are supposed to uphold the laws failed to do so, and the doctors who could have limited the damage looked the other way.

One reason for writing this book is to inform other traffic casualties and warn them of the pitfalls they may face following a serious accident. I want to prevent the 6,000 traffic casualties confronted with brain injury each year in the Netherlands from being treated the same way I was, medically, legally and socially.

At the same time, I want to speak to others suffering from non-congenital brain injury, and to their friends and family as well. According to the Netherlands Brain Foundation an estimated 85,000 persons in the Netherlands fall victim to brain injury as a result of (traffic) accidents or acts of violence every year. Until it strikes, most people in the victim's environment know nothing about brain injury at all. And even afterwards, onlookers have a hard time imagining what is actually happening and what the victim is going through.

In the bookstores, I found the subject conspicuous by its absence. This is not so strange. Usually, the patients themselves cannot write about it. Their brains have been injured, making it hard to think. Planning and keeping track of virtually any situation has become impossible for them, let alone talking, reading and writing about their experiences. People with brain injury lose such skills immediately, and sometimes only recover them to a certain extent after years of endless practice and perseverance. In addition, brain injury also causes problems with mobility and balance.

And all that time, not only is the bruised brain incapable of putting a book together, it can't even imagine that a book could be written on the subject.

The reader may now be wondering how I, a victim of brain injury, nonetheless managed to write this book. That is a good question. In the beginning, it was totally impossible for me. After my accident, it took me a year and a half before I could begin to write, at first just short paragraphs in a notebook. Only much later did I start making notes on my computer, which ultimately resulted in this book.

My primary goal in making notes was simply to learn to write and type again. In addition, I was also motivated by the awareness that I kept forgetting everything I thought and experienced. I realized that by writing things down I could at least re-read what I had written from time to time, and thus show myself I was making progress.

Moreover, writing offered a new way of communicating with my overburdened husband. As I will soon describe, talking and reasoning became virtually impossible for me in the immediate aftermath of my accident. Writing became a necessity.

The idea of writing for a wider public only occurred to me later. It would be a shame, I thought, if people in my situation continued to be unaware of what lies in store for them.

I still had no idea then that writing would be such a Sisyphean task for my bruised head. I calculated that I could finish the book in ten years at my speed. That seemed feasible. But I soon realized that I would never succeed without help from many people. 'True power is found in silence', wrote Jan and Trude at the time. Thanks to them, I was able to write and take walks in absolute silence during my recovery. Once a week, I had the run of their waterside house, a healing, loving gesture.

Also, this book would never have been completed on schedule without the help of Maggie Oattes, who showed me an easy way to color-code my growing files and make them accessible. Later, she even took over the job of keeping them up to date, a chaotic task for me. This way of organizing all the events related to my accident made it possible for me to reconstruct the black hole into which I had fallen and generated lists of dates to help jog my memory while writing. Moreover, for the first chapter, in which I reconstruct my stay in the hospital, I could make use of a number of written sources, such as hospital brochures, letters and cards I received, and my medical file with reports from nurses and doctors. Finally, there were many books and articles I mined for information.

Last but not least, my contacts with the outside world could never have had any real success if my husband, Willem Vrakking, had not given me such unqualified support in looking after my external affairs. It was he who encouraged me again and again to keep on writing. And now, already weighed down by his role as witness for the prosecution and fellow victim of my accident, he will also be exposed to what might be called literary victimization through this book.

Run Over

According to the weather report, Sunday, October 14, was a 'lovely, calm fall day' in my town. That morning, I had shown my husband the thank-you note I wanted to send to the friends, family, neighbors and colleagues who had given me so much support after a serious eye operation. I had an appointment with Müller Söhne, a firm in Wiesbaden, Germany, for the manufacture of a custom-made, hand-blown glass eye, the ultimate in artificial eyes. But this appointment had to be postponed, for immediately after mailing my letters I was knocked off my bicycle by a moped.

Ironically, everyone found a letter from me that Monday announcing I was in great shape, yet at the very same time I was lying unconscious with a brain contusion in the Medium Intensive Care Unit (MICU) of the University Hospital.

I later heard that the moped rider, F.H., aged 21, had taken the curve too wide and too fast and crashed into me head on.

Apparently, a shrieking ambulance rushed me unconscious to the hospital. There, the diagnosis was pronounced: brain injury, contusio cerebri.

The bill we later received, amounting to 284 Euros and 40 cents, stated that 23 kilometers had been covered during that ten-minute ride.

My bicycle was declared a total loss.

Following the head-on collision, two police officers went to inform my sons. Maarten, the oldest, was busy washing my car. Joost had just gotten up. Maarten lost his head completely. Joost seemed to react more coolly. Together they drove to the University Hospital, where scans, EEGs and x-rays were being made of their unconscious mother's brain, along with x-rays of her broken or badly bruised face, chest and other parts of the body.

Much of what happened there is a blank to me, but I have been able to reconstruct the following. White coats stand in a circle around my bed. One white coat on the right steps forward and speaks. Vaguely I make out a mop of curly hair. I am being asked a question.

Apparently they expect an answer. With difficulty, I say: 'Hospital'.

Is that my voice?

Now they want to know which hospital.

I answer, correctly: 'The UH'.

Indicating what these letters stand for is more difficult. In fact, it is beyond my capacity. For the first time in my life, my precious brain and head are letting me down. I feel as if I must take a university examination without having opened a single book.

Most likely, the white coats have failed to grasp this. Even I realize only much later that I am not my normal self. I can't even tell you what day it is. But I do tell anyone willing to listen that my short-term memory is on the blink.

Is there anyone who shares this opinion?

What questions am I supposed to ask, actually, and to whom?

I ask Willem what's wrong with me and he mumbles something about very severe concussion.

One benefit of a poorly functioning short-term memory is that I am totally unconcerned about my health.

Each snippet of information I get on the subject melts away in no time like snow in the sun.

Monday afternoon, on waking for a moment in my room in the neurology/trauma ward, I can no longer remember anything about the accident, not the ambulance, nor the emergency room, nor the MICU. All I want to know is: How did I get here? Was I mugged on the street?

Where is everybody?

The first stimuli from the environment to spur me to action are the questions from the neurologists. I am anxious to answer those questions well.

Willem brings my diary and a pen so that I can note everything down, including who comes to visit me on which day.

By repeating the name of the day a few times aloud, I can manage to remember what day it is. For the time being, this is the only 'action' I am capable of.

I probably forget to write things down. Often, I can't find my diary and pen, or I forget about their existence entirely.

Two days after the accident, it begins to dawn on me that something is terribly wrong with my brain. Joost writes in my diary that I was discharged from the Medium Intensive Care Unit yesterday and that scans and x-rays were made.

I remember nothing.

He is surprised to have to write this down for me because I can't find yesterday in my diary. But if you don't know what day today is, you don't know what day yesterday was either.

I try to write down the names of my visitors. It astounds me to hear that my two beloved aunts from North Holland came to see me. I can't remember anything about it.

I'm told that when they asked how the accident happened, I mumbled that they'd have to ask Willem.

I am in terrible pain and shivering with cold.

I can vaguely remember that someone wanted to examine my eyes today. I see the silhouette of a familiar eye doctor, but I can't think and soon nod off again.

Doctors are probably trained to talk to brain-damaged patients in a loud voice to make their words sink in. It works for awhile.

Now someone wants to look in my mouth. I can hardly get it open. Again I nod off.

I ask for our dentist because my mouth and jaw are so painful.

I get telephone calls during my stay in the hospital, but when I look in my diary I see only a couple of callers have been noted.

I can make only minimum use of my battered brain.

When people give their names over the telephone, I do not react. After hearing a name, I search my memory desperately for a connection. But all I get is a short circuit.

If my caller provides a little background information ('I was in the tennis club'), my sluggish brain gets the time it needs to do the job. 'Yes of course!' I can finally say.

I speak very slowly too, although I am not aware of it myself.

When I hang up, I forget everything immediately, even the caller's name.

The world is very far away. People are very far from me. I feel no understanding or warmth, I feel only distance and cold.

No one touches me.

From a great distance, people try to contact me at what seem to be random moments in the morning or evening.

It takes me by surprise. I can't ask my questions because I forget I have questions to ask.

When there is only one visitor at a time, I apparently respond normally. At least, no one seems to notice anything odd.

Next to my bed stands a brown-skinned nurse radiating warmth. Her figure seems sculpted by Rodin. Her voice has a nut-brown timbre and her accent betrays her origin in some sunny, Caribbean land.

Where have I heard that voice before?

I don't know her, never met her before. But her voice sounds familiar.

She tells me that she took care of me yesterday in the neurological Medium Intensive Care Unit. Now she has just come by to take my temperature and pulse.

My dear, she says, what cold hands you have!

In no time she spreads a second cotton blanket on my bed.

There is some discussion about the treatment of my eyes. I tell her she has lovely eyes, large and almond-brown.

She smiles modestly, says I'm exaggerating.

I go a step further and say she has lovely features. What a sweet person.

Too bad I can't ask her more. She says she has to go back to the MICU and shakes my hand.

Is it possible that memory works selectively? The expression 'my dear' triggered a little opening in my bruised brain. 'My dear' goes together with the insertion of the catheter. She must have done that in the MICU. She was the one who explained what was going to happen and put me at ease.

Her voice is engraved in my memory, but I have completely forgotten her face.

Another nurse, young and petite, sticks her head around the corner. She shakes my hand and is truly surprised when I don't recognize her.

She says that she looked after me in the emergency room. 'Last Sunday!'

Nothing clicks. I don't know her.

She tells me I was ice-cold and couldn't stop shivering.

I tell her I had constant pain in my head and face.

That doesn't surprise her at all. My head is in terrible shape, she says.

I ask her what's wrong with me.

'A very, very severe concussion, a broken cheekbone and a peri-orbital hematoma', she says, and leaves it at that.

The nurse asks what I did before the accident. I answer with difficulty.

She looks at me with concern.

I ask how long it will take until I'm my old self again.

Do I embarrass her? Hopefully, I add: 'Next week? Two weeks from now?'

Her expression tells me I am too optimistic.

'I know what', I exclaim, 'let's say six weeks!'

She listens to me with a friendly smile. An uneasy feeling comes over me: it is much worse than I thought.

Why won't she answer my question?

The nurse says goodbye. Will I see her again?

Who put these cozy socks on my feet?

And who sent these lovely photos of my sons?

Something lying on the windowsill is making me very uneasy. I don't know what it is or where it came from. Who put it there? What's it for?

Some nameless object is lying there and it frightens me.

Is something wrong with my head or my broken eye socket?

Or both?

Why can't I see what it is?

To lessen the fear I get out of bed, an agony I only confront when there is really no other choice. I make my way to the windowsill, to the sinister object.

It turns out to be nothing more than a bit of litter left behind by a visitor.

Back in bed I have forgotten what it was. But the fear is over.

Suddenly a voice rings through the room: 'We don't want you walking to the toilet on your own'. The nurse is quite definite about it. 'From now on you ring for the bedpan.' She shows me the bed bell too.

Am I suddenly getting my period? But that can't be right! The nurse reassures me: 'That often happens after accidents.'

Because I am afraid of falling out of bed I ask the nurse for safety rails. I am rather disoriented and feel safer behind bars.

When I wake up I don't know where I am, several times a day.

At night I want a light left on in the corridor.

The lamp above my bed is broken. This is dreadfully disconcerting to me.

I check to see whether I can move my arms.
    While sitting in bed, I can also raise my legs.
    There are huge blue marks on my thighs, intensely painful.
    I remember something called eye-hand coordination and try to touch the tip of my nose with a finger.
    Bringing my two index fingers together also poses no insurmountable problems.
    I even manage to move all my fingers.

16

It makes me feel a lot less anxious.

Above my bed hangs a metal triangle on a leather strap. Quite soon I realize that this triangle is very handy for pulling myself up to a sitting position, when I want to drink something, for instance.

My chest hurts so much. Agonizing pain shoots right up through the maximum dose of paracetamol. I move as little as possible.

Someone comes to ask if I want to renew my TV subscription. I have to say how many more days I want to use it.

I say: 'As long as I'm lying here.' The question embarrasses me.

How long has that thing been sitting at the end of my bed? And how much longer will I have the pleasure of its company in the University Hospital?

I say: 'Better ask the nurse.'

Why do I actually have a television and a telephone in my room? Are they good stimuli when you're lying in bed on your own?

I have to fill in a list of what I want to eat.

A cheese sandwich on whole-wheat and a glass of buttermilk sounds good.

It takes a long time to find them on the list. All the sentences and words are dancing before my eyes.

When I try to read something, I immediately forget what I want to fill in.

It is an impossible task.

I eat because I want to get well, but it is all tasteless.

The neurology unit manager, formerly known as the head nurse, is a tall blonde young woman with a serious manner: this is a place of work.

Today I may leave my bed. Under her escort, I go to the toilet.

I am shocked when I look in the mirror. Am I that strange person with the swollen head and expressionless gaze?

The toilet is no fun at all. I can't manage to lower myself onto the seat in the normal way. It is more like an emergency landing, with a hard bump resonating terribly through my head as I finally land on the right spot.

Pushing triggers a fierce surge of pressure in my head. To tear the toilet paper from the roll I have to twist my neck back and to the side. It makes me dizzy, as if I was falling off the earth.

I move like a helpless, purposeless creature.

With the unit manager, I make my first little outing. It is hardly an unqualified success. 'Do you always have such trouble walking?' she asks, as she drags me along the corridor.

Walking suddenly seems such an exhausting activity.

I stop and say: 'I don't know how to get my legs moving any more.' I am closer to tears than laughter.

I am helped back to my room, where I collapse into an exhausted sleep.

Before my accident, I had just decided not to go with Willem to a congress in Prague. It was scheduled during the period when our youngest son would be taking his first set of final exams at high school. I stayed home when our eldest son took his exams and he did well. I think it is nice for the children if I stay home to keep things running smoothly during such times.

Willem was disappointed. But now nothing is going according to plan anyway. The roles have been reversed. After every exam, Joost cycles over to visit his mother in the hospital before going home. A fifteen-kilometer trip, even though I am not always aware of it.

He is shocked by what he discovers. His mother doesn't even know what day it is and writes with great difficulty, in an abominable scribble. She forgets practically everything he tells her and repeats herself endlessly.

Yet he makes a calm and resolute impression. A visit from him is a pleasure. He doesn't talk much. He listens, probably thinking: 'Something's wrong here! Is this my mother?'

My cousin visited me immediately after the accident in the neurological observation room. She writes a card: 'I was so sorry for you. You lay there all bruised and wounded and you were so terribly cold. Luckily those men of yours were full of concern for you. At one point, I even felt a kind of joy to see how tenderly Maarten stroked his mother's arm and hand. I don't know if you felt it, so that's why I'm telling you now.'

I didn't know I was lying there, I didn't know who was there with me, and so I am pleased with her report. It's one more piece in this still so chaotic puzzle.

I understand I had quite a few visitors on the day of the accident. Willem allowed a good many people to approach the bed where I lay, unconscious but audibly present. I had great difficulty breathing, and was very noisy about it.

There must have been a lot of hustle and bustle around my bed. Nurses coming and going to check my pulse, heart and catheter, visits from the neurologist, the eye doctor, and the dentist, and then of course Willem and my sons, along with my aunts and cousin.

Why did no one tell Willem that this might be too much of a good thing? That so many visitors are annoying to the nursing staff and disturbing to the patients.

What is the best thing for the patient? To be frequently pulled out of unconsciousness or allowed to enjoy total rest?

Perhaps hospital rules should only permit visits by immediate family to MICU patients. This really seems to bother me.

Every time my husband or sons come to visit, they are shocked when I ask them how I landed in the hospital. I forget the reason again and again. Reluctantly, they have now brought a copy of the newspaper report of my traffic accident.

The clipping is posted on the bulletin board in my room. That way, I can read what happened myself if I forget it again. Luckily, I don't forget to look at the bulletin board at such moments.

From the local newspaper:

Tuesday, October 16. Municipal police reports. Collisions.

On Sunday afternoon, October 14, a cyclist was injured on the square in a collision with a moped whose driver took the curve too wide. The cyclist was taken to the University Hospital.

Now the process of imprinting my accident on my memory can begin. Will the reason I am lying here gradually sink in?

I say the Lord's Prayer with the hospital priest. It gives me strength. It is familiar and soothing.

Suddenly my mother and brother are sitting next to my bed with their arms full of flowers. Mama looks worriedly at my heavily swollen face. The purple rings around my eyes are visibly upsetting her. How could such a thing happen to her daughter? Hans stands in front of the bulletin board. Shaking his head, he studies the sketch of the accident scene made by Maarten. 'Don't forget I've been to see you, now!' Mama implores as she leaves.

I sit on a chair under the shower. Helpful hands carefully wash my hair. 'Are you okay, Mrs. Willemsen?' The head nurse dabs my dizzy head dry. I like these little cleanups.

Femke comes to visit with some of our favorite ice cream. The treat oozes out of the cone and the right corner of my mouth onto the sheets. 'This is going to be a hell of a mess' I sigh, glancing helplessly around. 'Is it doing you any good?' asks Femke, meanwhile calmly putting Kleenex on the sticky spots. We enjoy the ice cream together. I complain about severe neck pain.

'You'll tell the neurologist, won't you?' she says.

I am too confused for that. I can't even remember a message, let alone pass it on.

I am tired and can no longer talk to Femke. Not that she expects me to talk, but I am just not used to so much attention.

When I go to the toilet, she sees that I have great difficulty keeping my balance. I am glad she doesn't mention it.

Sunday and not a soul in sight. Where are Willem and the boys? Is there a golf tournament or something?

I feel that Willem's visits are too seldom and too short. When I tell him so, he swears he comes every day.

I miss Willem so much. He can't pacify me with stories about how busy he is at work. He has never been able to sit still.

When he talks about his cancelled trip to Prague I get irritated. He seems completely oblivious to the severity of my condition.

It is not made clear to him in the hospital, either.

In great haste, a colleague is now preparing to present his lecture in Prague. A big relief for Willem.

In a long, loving letter, Camelia writes: 'After all these tribulations, the future can't bring you anything but happiness. I was so shocked when I heard about it from Willem, but I was also glad you suffered no permanent injury. You are such a strong person that you will surely overcome this as well.'

On the tenth day in the hospital, I note in my diary: '7.45 a.m. EEG'. My second outing.

22

'Can you go to the EEG on your own?' the unit nurse asks. Since I don't immediately say no, she explains the route to me. I forget it right away. I leave my room, but then what?

I see nothing around me. I walk through a gray, formless space.

Am I blind?

I see nothing.

The nurse no doubt notices my halting steps: 'Do you think you can walk there with help?'

Of course I can. But I don't realize that I have hardly walked anywhere yet.

I have never been easily alarmed. This time, too, I have overestimated myself.

'Maybe a wheelchair would be better?' the nurse asks.

I say 'No, I haven't broken my legs, have I? And I'm not paralyzed either. No, it's definitely not needed.'

A man from general services takes my arm. He shepherds me through the labyrinthine hospital and sits me down on a chair on another floor. I see stars and am glad when I get to lie down for the EEG a little later.

The nurse smears my head, or actually my hair, with gunk from a tube, connects some electrical equipment, and goes to sit behind a glass partition. I see some brain waves registering on a little screen. What luck, there is still some life in my brain!

The nurse chats about her little boy and I chat back.

She says nothing about the EEG results.

I am planted back down on the chair in the hall to wait for the man in blue.

He doesn't come.

Now the mist around me is becoming truly impenetrable. I break out into a cold sweat.

I sigh more and more deeply, and everything goes black. I hear quick footsteps, people and nurses running. 'Are you okay, ma'am?'

I want to go to bed, I have trouble sitting up, waiting endlessly for my escort.

Since I keep sighing and don't respond to their questions, the other waiting patients, concerned about my moaning and groaning, call for help. I have never sat up so long before.

An arm appears, a man who finally takes me, walking again, back to my room.

Dead tired and totally disoriented, I collapse onto the bed and into sleep, still in my bathrobe.

In the neurology ward of the University Hospital, the doctors make their daily rounds between 8.30 and 9.30 in the morning. But I have been here nearly two weeks now and have only two vague memories of such visits. Have all their visits been clumped together into these two memories?

The idea of anticipating their visits, for instance by making sure I am lying there neatly washed and ironed when the doctors come by, has not even occurred to my bruised brain. They appear suddenly out of thin air, and as suddenly disappear again.

Although never in my life have I felt so miserable and dead tired, the doctors have decided that after eleven days in the hospital I can be discharged. The white coats come right up to my bed to tell me the news. I extend my hand to introduce myself, but one of the coats says I have already done that.

Most of his words go in one ear and out the other, because I am racking my brain to try to remember when I saw him before.

A few fragments of our conversation remain: '...if I was home, I wouldn't be good for much...if I could have help...home help...I can't be left on my own...'

I ask the doctor again who he is. On that Tuesday, October 23, I write his name in wobbly letters in my diary.

Once he knows I'm coming home, Willem wants to pick me up on Thursday instead of Friday or Saturday as agreed. Thursday is the only free day in his chockfull schedule.

Has he actually been told that I am still disoriented in time and have so much to endure?

Sunday's Child

When I leave the hospital, I have lost eight kilos, a pleasant side effect. Once I am home, my family doctor visits me every week. When his third visit approaches, thinking ahead for the first time, I have an important question for him. For safety's sake, I have written it down on a scrap of paper.

"Doctor, what's wrong with me?"

I have a notepad all ready and write with great difficulty in my still faltering scribble, the tip of my tongue protruding from my mouth: "brain bruise, comptusion?".

The doctor doesn't know what's happening to him. Is this Andrea Willemsen? But she must be in really bad shape. He asks: "Haven't you talked with the neurologist about this?" Not that I can remember. Didn't I get a letter from the treating neurologist? Haven't seen any letter. He promises to bring the letter next time.

I ask Willem if he has had a talk with the neurologist or read his letter to our doctor. No, he doesn't know anything about it either. When I persist, he tries to evade my reproaches.

He keeps silent as the tomb. I make no further progress. In any case, none of this is his fault.

I feel a strong sense of resistance well up inside me. What is going on here? Don't I have what it takes to handle my own affairs? And why won't anyone help me? I want to know what is wrong with me. And why no one has told the people closest to me.

I am also disappointed in Willem. How can he let his wife be discharged from the hospital without knowing exactly what is wrong with her? He must have his own ideas about it, but I can't tell what he's thinking from his expression.

Thoughts whirl and tumble through my head, causing enormous pressure in my skull. I feel desperate, powerless and alone, and in no shape to order anyone around. My head is failing me, I am brainless, decapitated. I have to go to bed.

The family doctor comes, produces the neurologist's letter from his bag and gives it to me to read. I force myself to seize the opportunity, but the letters are all dancing before my eyes. I don't manage to finish the task while he waits for me. I give the letter back, as if I know what's in it.

"Yes", says the doctor, "it doesn't say much more than that you should rest."

Rest. Now that was the one word I did manage to make out.

My rattled brain can't comprehend it all. Did I ask for a copy of the letter so that I could read it again in peace? In any case, I am in no shape to undertake the trek to the copy machine.

Later, maybe later, when I feel better, I think helplessly.

But what exactly is wrong with me?

Later, my experiences during those first weeks got me thinking about medical care in the Netherlands. My parents took very good care of me throughout my childhood and raised me lovingly. They always gave me the benefit of the best medical care. If a higher level of eye surgery was available in Utrecht than in Amsterdam, then neither expense nor trouble was spared to have my congenital cataract and squint operated on there by Professor of Ophthalmology Weve. In the early 1950s that was still quite a journey, by tram, train and on foot from Amsterdam to Utrecht and back. But it was more than worth the trouble. After the operation I looked a lot better, which was very important for the giggly girl my parents thought I was.

Following my most recent treatment I have less reason to be thankful. Can it be that I am the first brain-bruised traffic casualty to be treated in the University Hospital? And why is the communication with my husband and me so abominable? If I am not the first case of brain injury, then the neurologists must know by now what something like this can trigger in the victims. After my accident, the care provided by the doctors is seriously deficient, and I notice no effort at all, neither verbally nor in writing, to explain to us what might be going on.

Since I can no longer telephone, the first step towards a solution must come from the bookcase. Two old medical encyclopedias will have to do the trick. For a half an hour each day, I set to work on the index with a felt pen and a ruler, resulting in a page full of notes.

I write: "Brain contusion (contusio cerebri), serious injury to the brain, caused by external violence created and characterized by the symptoms of concussion and possible permanent disorders due to local damage to the brain tissue."

And: "Concussion, damage to the brain caused by external violence (a blow to the skull, a fall, etc.) without damage to the brain matter itself (commotio cerebri)."

Why am I so disregarded? In university hospitals, as I later come to understand, there are often so-called Medium

Intensive Care neurology wards for emergency cases, particularly traffic casualties. There are reasons for setting up separate wards for such cases. In general, the usual intensive care ward is used for operations on patients with heart and neurological problems, not incidentally areas which score high at medical congresses and in the international journals where doctors like to display their tours de force. Now and then you see them on television programs, where they trot out their latest medical miracles and show that even specialists are friendly folk with the best interests of their patients at heart. Frequently, exceptional cases are involved, amazing the audience and causing a sensation, and convincing the public of the great importance of the work of the medical profession.

But even a specialist has only two hands and one head. And as long as his attention is devoted to medical tours de force, not only will all his energy be focused there, but a great deal of his budget as well. Fine, he works hard, he has a right to perform, but the fact is that few neurologists, neurosurgeons and trauma specialists are interested in a phenomenon like brain contusion, let alone make any attempt to exchange data on the subject internationally.

In the medical world, the kind of brain injury I have is an unwanted child, the black sheep of the family. And the fact that this black sheep usually presents itself to healthcare workers at night or in the weekends doesn't make it any more popular.

Meanwhile, I have learned that there is a much better method of detecting acute brain injury ('closed head injury') than the summary examination carried out by the University Hospital following my accident. This better method is known as an MRI examination. What I have been asking myself since this discovery is why this technique was denied me at the crucial moment. Why, as a traffic casualty, was I not immediately offered the best examination technique available? The hospital had every modern screening technique for such examinations at its disposal, but when it came to using them, forget it! The costly equipment was left unutilized on the ward on that ill-fated day, while I just lay there, unconscious and incapable of either wanting or demanding anything.

Since then, there are more questions I find impossible to dismiss.

Surely, a hospital should know that an unconscious traffic casualty, run over through no fault of her own by a motorized oncoming driver, must be given an additional examination, if only to pinpoint the brain injury. Why was this not done? Was there no one to run the equipment on the day of my accident?

Is there some kind of 'never on Sunday' policy for MRIs?

And why were the so-called CT scans made only on the day after my accident? And where are those scans, anyway? Later, the hospital did its very best to try to find them, but, to my desperation, they are still irretrievably lost. Why was no thought given to the fact that injuries are often much less visible on the type of brain scans used for me? With a bit of pushing, anyone a little worried about his back can get a whole series of scans and x-rays made, often travelling to the University Hospital especially for that purpose. But to me the absolutely essential was denied.

Later I wonder whether my case may have been taken less seriously because I am a woman. I receive a newspaper clipping in which Prof. Dunning writes that medical examination facilities are frequently used in a very unequal manner, and that women are the main victims of this inequality. Following Bernadine Healy, Dunning calls this the 'Yentl syndrome'.

Was I a victim of that syndrome?

The question presents itself as to how, after such meager care, traffic casualties can be expected to arm themselves against the second wave of violence which may wash over them: that of the Other Party, the perpetrator's insurance company. Simply to defend themselves, victims should at least have proof of the damage available. You can just imagine what the insurance company experts will have to say on the subject: 'Gosh, ma'am, there weren't even MRIs made, so it can't be all that bad! I advise you to go through a course of psychological treatment, help you work a few things out for yourself, you'll see how much better you feel!'

Initially I assumed that my ailments and bumps would gradually disappear. But that's where I was mistaken. Three months after my accident I still have yellow spots under my eyes and my face is still completely stiff. Both my thighs display large yellow spots as well. Not to mention the pain I undergo and the great restrictions on movement.

And questions keep coming up. Why are no periodic examinations held to keep track of recovery in an injury to the brain and face? That's the least you would expect for someone who became unconscious through no fault of her own.

Slowly, the reality of what I am facing begins to sink in. Autopsies of patients who died from the type of 'closed head injury' I have suffered (yes, it can kill you!) reveal that the injuries can lead to loss of brain tissue. I begin to be terribly worried. What will it be like when I'm a little older? Have I reason to be more anxious than other people? The neurologist denies this most decidedly, but I fear it is true.

According to Dr. R. Braakman, a former professor of neurosurgery who has visited most of the neurosurgical centers in the Netherlands as a member of the inspection committee, my case is no exception: neurosurgical procedures are regularly violated. In his farewell lecture , he will state that the desired sequence of examination for patients suffering disorders of consciousness following (traffic) accidents should be as follows: first, an x-ray of the skull. Then, if there is a skull fracture, a computerized tomography scan (CT scan) of the brain must be carried out as soon as possible. If the patient is in coma, Braakman states that this examination must be carried out with the greatest possible speed in a neurosurgical center.

In retrospect, reconstructing what happened to me following that disastrous accident, I come to understand that I could not have had it worse. I was a woman, unconscious through no fault of her own, brought it on Sunday and, on top of it all, treated by an intern who ignored the guidelines.

In my medical report, neurologists and nurses observe that I am 'confused' and have 'anterograde amnesia', combined with 'disorientation in space and time'. Why then, I wonder, has no one reacted to this? And why did I immediately have to act as my own spokeswoman to my husband and two sons? It seems like a really sick joke. Later, Willem tells me he heard nothing about the scale of my limitations, neither from the neurologists nor from the nursing staff.

Only during a long drive, when he can no longer evade discussion of the topic, does Willem tell me that, when it all started, he called our family doctor a number of times to ask about my situation. He came away little the wiser for it.

If only Willem had contacted the treating neurologist himself immediately, or in any case when I was discharged from the hospital. But instead he called his doctor to seek support, to cope with the fact that he had come out of the accident without a scratch, while I took the full blast. Willem was of course much too upset himself to wonder how things were going with me.

Written Off

Only in early November, weeks after the accident, do I first hear the official medical diagnosis of what has happened to me: I am suffering from 'diffuse brain injury'. What that precisely means to me and my family is already quite clear to me. A burning forehead, pain in my face, in my back and neck vertebrae, in my left hand and in my right hip.

I have had to adapt my daily schedule and activities, for I have no more than two hours worth of energy available each day. In the course of the day there is increasing pressure on my skull, ears, forehead, eyebrows and nose, and I have great difficulty getting through the weekends with their unexpected visits. Chatting with the children when they come home demands so much energy that I have to leave the shopping and cooking to Willem. What I like best is to withdraw to a quiet room to get a bit of peace.

That withdrawal is essential. If I neglect it, I am sure to have a seriously restless night. And there are more things from which I need to retreat. I have come to hate telephone calls. All my sports have been abandoned by now: no more golf, no tennis, no fitness training, hikes in the mountains, skiing, skating or swimming. And no concerts or museums either.

Not only have all my daily social contacts been cancelled, but my professional and scientific contacts have also been cut off outright. I have had to stop all my paid and unpaid work. No longer can I work as an administrative researcher and consultant. No more research on my dissertation. No more working for my political party either, where I used to be a member of the traffic work group. Everything is gone.

I feel that I have been written off.

Exactly four weeks after my discharge from the University Hospital, I have an appointment for a check-up at the neurological outpatient clinic. My medical file reports the reasons: trauma capitis, left zygomatic fracture, light to moderate diffuse brain injury with a few hours of posttraumatic amnesia.

To be sure that we don't forget anything, Willem and I have submitted a written list of questions in advance.

Two doctors in white coats sit down across from us. The intern takes the floor. She remarks that I have a lot of questions.

Due to pain in my left eye when looking down, I am referred to the eye clinic. I have also reported that my vision is blurry. With the greatest difficulty, I can manage to decipher the biggest headline in the morning paper. It takes a lot of time and is such a terrible effort that I quickly halted the experiment. Everything wiggles and jiggles in front of my eyes. I simply can't see the letters straight.

But most of the questions on our list remain unanswered. After the talk, Willem and I go home again with empty hands. We don't get it at all. Is the young doctor not supposed to say anything because she is only an intern? We are little or none the wiser about the examination techniques used in my case. We don't blame the intern for this, but we are nonetheless disappointed to have received so little information in response to our carefully prepared questions.

Despite the fact that I feel completely broken down, I am treated as though I was 'unaffected'. What is going on here? Are the doctors taking my complaints too lightly? Have they any notion at all of my zombie-like existence? They do not encourage a great deal of exercise, but relaxation exercises led by a physiotherapist, they tell me, would be good for me. Although I have never felt so 'headless' as I do now, the doctor has the nerve to tell me that rest is the only way to relieve my complaints.

To say that I feel 'somewhat muddled' is definitely a very subtle description of the fact that I can hardly think straight. Making coffee has become a time-consuming and complicated chore. Is that why the doctors describe my concentration as 'not yet optimum'?

I am despondent. How can I ever reach my old level again when the least effort creates this enormous feeling of pressure in my head? I can't read for long at all. I succeed in comprehending the content only with the greatest effort. This is also what the neurologist has written to our family doctor and the ophthalmologist. So why am I not referred somewhere to find out what is so very wrong with me and how to make it better?

It seems nobody is aware of what I am going through. My complaints about fierce pain in my neck and back vertebrae are not pursued. No physiotherapy or manual therapy is proposed to ease my stiff face and forehead. The disappearance of my sense of smell and taste is ignored. Apparently, my complaints are no cause of concern to anyone and appear quite in keeping with the injury I have suffered.

Meanwhile, my reality has become unlivable and unworkable. How long can a person exist like this?

By now I also have a great deal of pain in my nose, cheeks and jaw. That is not so surprising when a moped rider wearing a helmet has bored head-on into your face like a projectile at 40 km per hour. In any case, three months after the accident the first abscess presented itself. Like a goofy drunk, I am delivered to the dentist, who, after an incision to relieve the pain, refers me to the periodontic surgeon. Since I am neither physically nor psychologically capable of enduring a long operation to save the molar, I choose to have it pulled out, partly because of the operation's success rate of only 20 to 40%.

So back I go to the dentist who, as a neighbor, offers to plan the appointments so that I can ride with him to his office. He at least sees the state I am in.

I have great difficulty climbing the steps to his office. Agonizingly slow, with both hands on the banisters. An eighty-year-old woman could do it faster.

Once in his office I don't say much. After the treatment I have to sit quietly on the chair for a long time, because trying to get up makes me dizzy. When I finally go down the stairs again, he keeps an eye on me. 'Are you okay?' No, not really.

But it can always get worse. My jaw also appears to have been damaged in the accident, with the result that I no longer have a good bite (occlusion). I can no longer put my teeth together and can hardly eat. Based on the x-rays, my dentist concludes with amazement that my jaw has been permanently dislocated and he treats me for fourteen long sessions. He first repairs the bite. To my horror, he must grind down my beautiful front teeth for this purpose. I look on sadly, aware that I have no choice—at least if I want to chew normally again. Finally he builds me a new bridge with his skillful hands.

Christmas

After the accident, my family life changed from one minute to the next. Each year around Christmas, the whole family usually heads up to the snow country. But as the holidays approach, two months after my accident, plates are falling out of my hands at home, not only because I am in the clumsy ('butterfingers') phase, but also out of pure frustration. I feel terribly angry. Angry, because nobody helps me clear the table, while it is obvious I can't do it on my own. Angry, because nobody understands what is going on with me, and I have absolutely no idea myself. Angry, because nobody listens to me, and I'm not used to that.

Am I no longer so convincing, do I sometimes talk nonsense, am I inconsistent? No, of course not. I am simply torn between wanting to do my duty and wondering why everything is now so impossible for me.

Why else should I be surprised when my unquestionably hard-working husband lets me know in December that he thinks I can easily come along to our place in the snow? 'Don't be so nervous! No problem! You feel awful here, maybe it will be better up there, in the sunshine.' That's the line he takes.

But I can't think things through in my condition, let alone put what I feel and want into words. I cry, no, I scream, exasperated that none of them understands anything, and smash the pile of plates I'm clearing up onto the floor.

A deathly silence follows.

That has never happened before, Mother smashing plates and obviously completely upset. My sons look at me with amazement and horror.

Then they all try to calm me down. But meanwhile they stick to their guns. They don't see a single reason for staying home at Christmas. They will take care of everything for me. I won't have to worry about anything.

But all I want is to be consoled. I feel like such a miserable zombie. My poor head practically bursts from the pressure when I try to think and express myself. It keeps my lips sealed, and anyway I can't find the right words. What is this all about? My voice falters when I try to speak and I know that this will only pass with rest and solitude.

I feel no panic, only impotence.

Deep in my heart I know I just want to stay home. Finally I find the words to say so, but they are politely brushed aside, as if I had made a suggestion too foolish for words. Who will cook for me then, who will help me with all the unforeseen things I simply cannot do for myself? But I don't at all wish to be separated from the people who are dearest to me on earth. The only thing I want is to be close to my family, and they are going to the mountains.

Finally, this feeling proves to be decisive. I follow my heart and land in an impossible situation. The snowball begins to roll, triggering an avalanche of problems.

Neither the neurologist nor the family doctor foresee any problems with my trip, they say, provided I take enough rest.

No problem, we think. At my request, the doctor has arranged a wheelchair for me at the airport, a necessity in the busy Christmas season due to my problems with balance and walking. Everyone agrees that a change of scene will do me good. Let her enjoy herself!

I ask my oldest son, a student in Delft, whether I have a greater chance of cerebral hemorrhage or stroke by going up to 2000 meters with my contusio cerebri. He sends me a loving letter with a short lecture on the difference in air pressure between Holland and the Alps. He does not expect a pressure difference of some 100 to 200 millibars to cause internal bleeding. He assumes that internal bleeding due to low air pressure is much less likely than external bleeding, since the blood vessels on the surface of the body actually 'feel' the reduction in counterpressure. It is known, he writes, that bloody noses and small wounds heal slowly at very great heights (8000 m) due to low air pressure, but at 2000 meters this difference is negligible.

There is another difference between the lowlands by the sea and the high mountains, he tells me. In the Netherlands, the oxygen content of the air is normally around 20%, while in the Alps it is less. But even that should be no problem, according to my son. 'The feeling of thin air and breathlessness is caused by a lower oxygen level', he writes. A body unaccustomed to low-oxygen air will have to adapt. At 2000 meters, to acquire as much energy as in Holland puts a heavier burden on heart and lungs. He concludes his advice by saying that further thought and verification are called for here.

Wonderful, to have a son who not only helps me think, but also wants me to just come along 'as usual'.

Naturally, the trip produces major problems right from the start. The airport is full to bursting at Christmastime. Despite my wheelchair, the journey will be a heavy burden for me. My son Joost, just 17, will travel with me while Willem and my other son, Maarten, make the trip by car. That way we won't have to lug so much baggage along. I also have the most confidence in Joost, because while I was bedridden after the accident he was with me almost daily. He cooked and cared for me. Of the three of them, he is the most aware of my misery.

But he is also the youngest. At one point, when he pushes the wheelchair too quickly and turns too abruptly, I snap at him. I have become dizzy and can no longer see my hand before my eyes.

I can't stand the jolting of the wheelchair. My brains seem to be sloshing around in my head. Each time he speeds up or slows down, no matter how slightly, all my brain cells slide forwards or backwards. My body's suspension system, which should ensure that my head, neck and back absorb shocks, appears to be terribly defective. My shock absorbers have broken down, causing me great pain.

The first hour of the trip I manage to behave like a big girl, but then melancholy takes over. I hang my head, no longer able to sit up straight, in an ever-increasing sprawl. I have only one desire: to lie down.

I don't know yet that the combination of lying down and silence is the main requirement for recovery. The train trip, a total of three hours through the mountains, including changing trains twice, leaning on Joost's arm, waiting on packed platforms, no reserved seats, to make matters worse it was a local, and hordes of passengers getting on and off the crowded second-class car, my fellow travelers eating and crackling their newspapers, whining children, people talking—for me it is a journey through hell.

Joost has a heavy responsibility on his shoulders. He must stay with me at all times, even accompanying me to the toilet. I am so dead tired that I can't find my way in all these unfamiliar spaces.

I see everything through a haze. And my nerves are completely on edge. Keep your eyes open, Joost, make sure the timings haven't changed. I can't stand any more surprises. I know that surprises mean delay and I want only one thing: to go to bed and close my eyes.

When we finally arrive at 2000 meters, Joost and I get into a horse-drawn sleigh as usual. But what a horror this turns out to be. After only twenty meters I have to get down again. I can't bear the driver jerking at the reins and the uneven pace of the trotting horses. A couple of times, when the horses suddenly sink into the deep snow, I practically scream with pain. There is nothing for it but to walk the rest of the way.

In the apartment, Joost makes my bed and tells me, 'Sleep well now, Mama'. And then the problems start up again. Hubbub on the attic stairs, the noisy front door, heavy shoes, racket on the bedroom stairs, noise from downstairs and the open kitchen, the sounds of the television and my husband and sons talking and laughing together.

This, I decide, is my last time in this apartment.

The next day, I ask Willem to buy five postcards to send to our nearest and dearest. But he thinks it grossly exaggerated to have to write them for me too. He thinks I can do it perfectly well myself. I know what it means, though. And, indeed, again and again I lose track of the addresses I am trying to copy from the paper in front of me. I can't see them clearly. I make spelling mistakes. I can't remember the words and their place on the page and their spelling. It is an impossible task. For a long time I try my best, until finally Willem grudgingly takes over. Do we really have to send cards everywhere? 'If you can't handle it, don't do it!'

I confine myself to writing 'best regards' and our names on the cards. With the word 'best' I forget the 's'. The word looks strange to me anyway. Shouldn't it have an 'a' instead of an 'e'? Later, my godmother will ask whether it was me who wrote that card. She could not recognize the trembling, straggly handwriting.

After writing the cards I am so exhausted I must go and lie down. I won't try it again anytime soon. I have asked too much of myself. But how else was I supposed to know whether I could do it or not, maybe even effortlessly?

On the return journey we again have to travel three hours by train. I arrive at the airport with my head hanging down, like a broken reed. We run into a neighbor who has not yet heard what happened to me. I explain. At the end I am totally debilitated and say that I don't want to see anyone any more. 'Throw a cloth over the wheelchair. I'm gone.'

Joost doesn't lose patience and says, chiding me slightly: 'Just don't say anything, Mom.'

Yes, if it were only that simple.

Neurological Patient

Five months after the accident a new and rather acute problem manifests itself. The production of speech, not merely in the sense of finding the right words, but the actual pronunciation and articulation, gives me so much pain and takes so much effort that I no longer answer the telephone and refuse all visits.

Moreover, any contact produces such extreme irritation and chemical reaction in my brain that I am completely out of circulation in no time. I am aware that everyone gathers data from different parts of the memory, compiles and evaluates them and then expresses the result, but I had no idea that this skill can be so exhausting. Formerly, I could always count on enormous energy, but now each stimulus produced by voice or machine is a torment.

I write down all these complaints in a six-page letter to the neurologist and ask Willem to make an appointment with him. On the day of the appointment we go to him together. There is no other way. Once I have managed to get my feet moving, I can usually no longer keep my eyes open, so a strong arm is no superfluous luxury.

Meanwhile, my considerate husband has greatly enlarged all the letters on my list, so I will be able to read them again with the help of a ruler. The letter concludes with a list of points that have improved, including the approximate dates on which various symptoms disappeared. I want to show that I consider each step forward, no matter how small, as a positive development. And also, since I do not yet have much insight into what is wrong with me and how I am going to recover, it seems to make sense to note down each instance of recovery in any case, no matter how much trouble and effort it takes. What is more encouraging than to look at areas where progress is being made? Besides, it must be no fun for a neurologist to always have to go through long lists of complaints. Anyway, I think my letter should end on a positive note.

So there I sit, full of hope that the doctor can improve my situation or in any case reduce the pain. I still have the greatest confidence in him, without having any idea if it is justified or not.

I ask him what is meant by diffuse brain injury and whether he can indicate which parts of the brain were affected. 'No', he says, 'with diffuse brain injury it is impossible to determine which areas are involved. The so-called black hole that can occur following the injury is known as posttraumatic amnesia or PTA. In your case, this has been established at one to two days. The scans show no damage to nerve cells. Fortunately, there are no pulpy spots to be seen.

The fact that this is good news does not immediately sink in, so the neurologist repeats it. We look blank. Later, we understand that 'pulpy spots' usually indicate what is known as failure. If there is no failure, the chance of recovery is very good.

However, we are told that the examinations carried out on me do not indicate whether I will completely recover, nor whether I will be subject to limitations. In any case, the neurologist does not believe that the head injury I have suffered will bring with it increased risk of brain diseases such as Alzheimer's in the long term.

He is unable to reassure me. Certainly not when I later read that head injury with loss of consciousness is indeed one of the risk factors for Alzheimer's disease. When I ask the neurologist where I stand, his advice is: 'Take rest, and practice a little on the computer every day.'

In short, nothing but generalizations. Despite all the energy I put into my letter, I am given no advice of any use to me. If only he had said, 'Madam, cases like yours, cyclists hit head on in the face and the breastbone by motor vehicles, are in the first place difficult patients for us to treat, patients whose complaints never cease. We don't even know where to begin with them, since we don't know which parts of the brain are involved. That's also why we call it diffuse brain injury.' But no. No sign of openness at all.

There is another thing I want to discuss with the neurologist. Since sports are out of the question for me for the time being, I am beginning to worry about my condition, my weakening and atrophying muscles and my cholesterol level. Before my accident, a strict diet and intensive exercise had enabled me to reduce my high cholesterol level to an acceptable maximum by Dutch standards. But how am I to stimulate better circulation and functioning in my heart, brain and legs now that even walking has become a problem?

When I ask about this, however, his answer is again disappointing. The art, I am told, is to inch forward bit by bit from now on. Over the next half year, the neurologist assures me, there may well be 'some improvement'.

One last point I put on my list, after talking with Willem, is that my sexuality has been affected. I have, as they say, lost interest. To tell the truth, it is far from easy for me to bring up such an intimate matter with the neurologist, but the differences between my sexual feelings before and after the accident are blatantly obvious. Before, as Willem used to say, I 'couldn't get enough of it'. Now it leaves me cold. I react to his advances with unmistakable repugnance. The look in my eyes tells him I've had more than enough before he even gets going. How can he even think about sex now? At such times, I feel completely taken off guard and see it as an invasion of my personal freedom. There is just no question of it for the time being.

My lack of interest in sex must have to do with my disturbed emotional life. Crying is alien to me, but now I become intensely emotional about certain things. I find my own behavior exaggerated and annoying at such times.

But this subject also appears to be taboo.

Two months after our visit, the neurologist writes to our family doctor: 'Patient is still having difficulty resuming her normal life and has provided a detailed written description of this.' Another appointment with him would serve no purpose, he says. Something tells me he thinks my complaints are exaggerated. This astonishes me.

The neurological treatment has come to an end. Apparently, my case is closed. I don't know what to make of this. I have no doubt that the neurologist, like many other neurologists, has a multicolored palette of patients with various types of brain problems to deal with. And of course some of these patients will have to come back for regular checkups. Certainly the patients on drugs will have to be seen by him at regular intervals. For them, at least, individual aftercare will have to be provided. But why does he leave patients with acquired brain injury who are not taking drugs in the cold? Why do I automatically get no more than a single piece of advice, namely to gradually increase the intensity of my activities? That may be plain speaking, but to my husband and me it is not plain enough.

On a beautiful day in May, still somewhat wobbly, I climb onto a bicycle for the first time by myself. I stay away for nearly a half-hour.

Joost wants to know exactly what route I plan to take. And even when he's not home, he insists that I write down when I leave and where I'm going. His concern is by no means odd. My ability to orient myself is still far from perfect. And imagine having to go off hunting for your mother.

Meanwhile my problems persist. I still have deficiencies on all fronts and am absent on all social occasions. My situation simply doesn't change, so Willem decides to again bring me to the attention of the treating— or formerly treating—neurologist. I make a new list of complaints, this time keeping it to a single sheet of paper. That may seem like a tremendous improvement, but where brain injury is concerned, nothing that can be put into words should be confused with reality.

For how many things can I still not feel, how much can I still not do? It is now fourteen months since the accident and I still have pain in my left eye and neck, I see poorly, feel burning spots on my head and face, have a jolting, uncontrolled walk, suffer from deafness, a lack of coordination when walking, experience severe physical and mental exhaustion and don't sleep well at night. On top of that I have trouble with my motor system, making it difficult to write or draw. I can't open cans, turn taps on and off, pour liquids from pans and walk against the wind.

And I'm still all thumbs, dropping and breaking things all the time.

By the time we see the neurologist, Willem has already contacted him a couple of times by phone. He also feels terribly weighed down by everything that has happened. Besides holding a part-time professorship, he runs an organizational consultancy with a few other people and now he has my brain trauma to deal with as well. I know I should be understanding and grateful for all his loving care on my behalf, but I can't keep myself from making light of his efforts. After all, wouldn't I do the same for him?

What I want to hear from the neurologist at our second visit is whether or not any real healing is in process. Does he have any idea of how serious the consequences of the accident are for me? I would also like to get as much information as possible about my injured brain. Where was it injured and how is the healing process progressing? Right after the accident I was incapable of doing the slightest thing for myself. I was totally unaware of the source of all my motor and cognitive defects. Yes, because of that damned accident, that was clear enough. But if you break your leg you get over it eventually, don't you? Anyone who has ever played hockey will be quite familiar with bruises, but they go away by themselves. When I used to play volleyball in high school I would bruise my fingers time and time again. It was no fun playing the piano afterwards, but there was no need to go the doctor. Why should it be different with bruised brains?

     True, my bruises in this case landed me in the hospital, but that was reasonable enough. After all, I was unconscious. I had ten to fourteen days of care, followed by a checkup with the specialist, and expected that that would be that. My medical treatment was more or less stopped, and if no more medical treatment was necessary, why shouldn't you just get better?

The list of questions I would like to ask seems endless. But despite all my lists of insurmountable problems, is there perhaps nothing more to treat? So am I cured then?

The second visit also ends with disappointment. I had hoped that when the neurologist saw my long inventory of complaints he would exclaim 'But Madam, why didn't you tell me sooner? We have first-rate drugs for all that!' Or that he would refer me to another expert who could intensify and supervise the healing process.

But once again, nothing of the kind. After our visit I am left on my own, with my 'odd' and 'painful' complaints. The neurologist nodded sympathetically during my monotonous litany, but what good does that do me? I get the feeling that he 'treats' people with similar complaints every day. Is it that he simply doesn't take me seriously, or does the impossibility of treating patients like me play a role? But then why doesn't he just say so?

How happy I would be if he had only referred me to someone who could guide me through this period, the most difficult of my life. And if he had just told me, 'Madam, we can do very little (i.e. nothing) for you.'

I feel left in the lurch. There is nothing to be done. The neurologist sees no need to make a new appointment. But how am I supposed to go on? Above all, I should rest as much as possible and build up my activities gradually. That is clear. But how do you do that with a bruised brain?

Next Time Stone Dead Please

When I regained consciousness after the accident, one of my first concerns was my eyesight. Did my good eye still work? My anxiety heightened as it gradually became clear that the big problems were with my brain. The combination of memory loss, ##anterograde amnesia and diminished eyesight did not seem very auspicious. My heart was in my mouth. Were my eyes actually examined? I have no clear recollection.

Once discharged from hospital, my eyes continued to be a growing source of complaint. And all these complaints were followed by advice from the ophthalmologists and eye surgeons. Then came two operations that unfortunately failed to produce the desired results. I still had high hopes that "they" would fix things up for me. But since my (painful) complaints continued to intensify, the surgeons proposed new and more radical operations.

I felt drained, at the end of my tether. I was even jealous of healthy people like Willem. What a luxury to have nothing wrong with you. I was fed up with all the medical treatments I had to go through. Sometimes I thought to myself in despair: if only I had been killed outright, then I would have been spared all this. Luckily these despairing thoughts did not get the better of me and I could usually push them away. In any case, I didn't have much choice: I was still alive.

Postponing the operations seemed like the only solution to me. The eye surgeon could always operate if things suddenly got worse. At first the ophthalmologists were against this idea, but I derived a great deal of satisfaction from the fact that I managed to drop out of the surgical merry-go-round. So it was possible after all.

During the winter one and a half years after the accident the amount of medical care I require reaches a record level. I have a season ticket to the University Hospital, a shoebox full of cards from various departments. That's the limit, I think to myself, both for Willem and me.

But the end is not yet in sight. A deluge of medical data from the hospital takes me by surprise. It breaks my spirit. If anyone so much as glances at me I burst into tears, although I've never been a crybaby. I feel totally stressed out, as does Willem, who has to bend over backward to keep me, the foundering wreck, on course. I am no longer capable of collecting information or reading it through, I can't even deal with it over the phone. Delegating is no longer possible, for the process of explaining and precisely formulating the questions to be asked is too complicated and exhausting for me. I feel powerless and don't know where to turn. My back's against the wall. The diagnosis of all my ailments and infirmities, I have come to believe, will only be complete when I am cut open from head to toe on the autopsy table.

Then come two lengthy, exhausting sessions during which I am tested by a neuropsychologist engaged by the moped rider's insurance company. I am happy that something like this is finally happening. The fact that I am obliged to submit to this test and by and for whom it is being done is not clear to me at first.

When it's over Willem tells me that according to Dutch disability criteria I am 100% incapacitated.

The verdict hits me hard. Six months after my accident, Willem and I read a short newspaper article about the Brain Foundation in Amersfoort and decided to attend one of their meetings. The foundation works with people with brain injuries, people like me. No lack of fellow-sufferers, evidently. When we arrived I found myself sitting around a table with people of my age who all turned out to be survivors of traffic accidents.

Now that I know what my future looks like, I think back on their stories. The man who sat next to me, a university professor, said that his wife had left him after the accident. He spoke in a slow monotone. He said he remembered nothing of the time he lay in coma. After a number of years, he now had a new girlfriend. But he would never work again. He visited his fitness club regularly.

This was the first time since my accident that I had taken part in a group discussion and I was eager to join in. I stood up, began to hold forth about what had happened to me, and suddenly lost the thread. No one thought it odd. But I shut up and sat down and thought, phew, so this is a problem too! How strange my voice sounded, choked up with emotions. And why did everything turn gray when I simply tried to concentrate on what I wanted to say?

Someone asked me why I kept holding my hands in front of my eyes or rubbing my head, leaning on my elbows for support. I replied: "I can't help it. I'm dead tired, my head feels like a ball of fire giving off incandescent sparks and I simply can't bear all these people, so I'm hiding myself."

I remember how much I wanted to get out of there. There were some plucky mothers who took the floor, determined to carve out a way in the world for their injured children, insisting that new ways of teaching be developed. But it just made my head spin. Any input was too much for me now.

On the way home Willem was obviously terribly moved. Was it because he saw how I floundered when I tried to speak, that he had seen with his own eyes how I fumbled for words, how unlike my old self I had become? No, it was because at the table where he sat that afternoon he was surrounded by wives whose husbands had suffered brain injuries. And he had just heard the most heartrending stories at this table of spouses. How the women looked after their husbands who were no longer the men they had married, and how their husbands' misfortunes had become life sentences for them as well.

It was enough to make you weep, said Willem. He still had no idea what our life would be like in the future.

The next time someone runs me over, I hope he finishes the job. Kill me stone dead please! Don't be a wimp about it and leave me again condemned to a brain injury.

When you have been lying unconscious for some time after a serious traffic accident, as soon as you come round everyone expects you to be happy you are still alive. But the strange thing about patients with brain injuries is that they are incapable of feeling any kind of happiness, let alone showing it. Means of expression such as crying, laughing and smiling are denied them.

The first few weeks after my accident I felt absolutely nothing. I was hardly participating in life at all. "Aren't you happy you can go home now?" No.

In the beginning I thought about death all the time, for I felt that I was dead. I found support in my faith, in a way it was even a sort of escape route for me. But there was no one I could talk to about death. I couldn't go to church for the same reason I couldn't go to concerts: too busy, too crowded, too noisy.

I also wanted to find out as much about death as possible. Since a superficial listener might easily interpret this wish as a sign of depression, a quite common phenomenon following a traffic accident resulting in brain injury, I thought it safer to keep my mouth shut. And the few people I did ask about it seemed taken aback. Furrowed brows: O God, now what! I gave them the creeps.

But the first ten months after the accident were a living hell. Like a brain-dead zombie I dragged my unmanageable body around the house. The only thing left of me was that body, driven not by an alert mind but by a motor system that seemed to have a mind of its own. Nothing was under my control. Only because I am what Willem calls a born optimist did I never feel the urge to take my own life in those days.

It was mainly the combination of a brain injury with the high frequency of operations scheduled for me and the decisions I had to make that caused my resistance to crumble away to almost nothing. Decision-making was no longer my strong point, what I had become good at was putting things off. Special courses are given to help people mourn their dead, but survivors of traffic accidents like me disappear into a big black hole. Why couldn't I sign up for a therapy to help me deal with the consequences of brain injury?

Almost two years after the accident I write in a notebook: This morning in the shower I was overcome by anxiety at the idea of having to grow old with this damaged brain. Old and dependent, how awful. And the worst thing is when the decision-making center, the brain, is out of order or only half-functional. I already have some experience of that now, at the age of 45, while women can easily live to 80. Life already consists to a great extent of suffering, surrender of independence and abdication of participation and communication. It is a sacrifice that is hardly bearable. After all, communication, both active (talking) and passive (active listening) is what distinguishes humans from animals

A Sheep on its Back

It is now two years since the accident. Once a week, I go to a summer house owned by friends. From my seat at the writing table, not only do I have a magnificent view of a pond set in a classic winter landscape, but it is also absolutely silent. The house is in a nature sanctuary where traffic is forbidden. Spending the day here is like a ray of sunshine in my otherwise dismal life.

I am inspired by a book called *Touching the Rock* by Prof. J.M. Hull who, when he became blind, also sought a peaceful spot in which to concentrate. He found it in the school where his sister taught.

Like Hull, I am brought here and picked up again each time. For the first time, I notice during these one-day hermitages that my headaches can be soothed by taking little walks. What a delightful discovery! Finally a straw I can clutch at.

At regular intervals I go out for a breath of fresh air. On one of my little outings I walk over the dike bordered on both sides by built-up fields. There, in the distance, among a herd of noisily grazing sheep, I see a sheep on its back, its feet in the air. I stop dead in my tracks and look again to make sure. My god, that poor sheep is totally motionless. It's just lying there stock-still with its legs pointing stiffly to the sky. What a pitiful sight! That sheep is in a coma. I must do something right now.

By coincidence, I read a newspaper article about this phenomenon not so long ago. A sheep on its back, or a 'cast sheep' as some farmers call it, is doomed to die in a couple of hours if nothing is done. Time to sound the alarm then.

Because of my problems with balance I can't save the victim myself. Moreover, there are several little ditches between the cast sheep and me. As quickly as my wobbly steps on the uneven dike permit, I hurry to the neighbor's house.

'There's a sheep on its back in the pasture!' I call out anxiously when the neighbor opens his door. He immediately phones the sheep's owner. The rescue can begin.

Then I see the connection between the sheep on its back and the unconscious, comatose traffic casualty. The accident victim also needs immediate rescue to limit the damage. With a sheep on its back, the assumption is that a displacement and twisting of its four stomachs has occurred, resulting in bacterial poisoning which, if emergency treatment is not given, will lead to death. Just like unconscious traffic casualties, such sheep must be helped to their feet again as quickly as possible and held firmly for some time until they can stand entirely on their own again. The only difference is that this process is somewhat more rapid in sheep than in people.

A week later, I hear that my sheep was saved from death at the very last moment.

My brain is out of balance. The transfer of electrical signals between the nerve cells in the brain is regulated by chemicals called neurotransmitters. My neurotransmitters are not doing their job. In my head, the swift switching mechanism, the nimbleness and maneuverability of my thoughts, has changed into a slow, clanking gearbox. I used to be a Porsche, but have now been downgraded to a Model T.

Before the accident I was a fluent speaker, never at a loss for words and adept in dealing with various topics in detail. If I was a novice in a field new to me, I knew I could count on my bilingual dictionaries, and my grammar books from high school also served me well. Until the accident. Since then, there has been a blackout in my capacity to absorb and process information.

Passive listening has always been foreign to me. I have an inquisitive nature. But active listening is an activity I can no longer sustain, for it gives me a throbbing headache. Passive listening would thus fit well with my new lifestyle. But am I supposed to just sit there like a couch potato and not take part? Would I be able to manage that? No. Conversation thrusts itself upon me, whether I like it or not. My brain reacts to whatever is being said. The fact that I don't need to say anything doesn't save me much energy.

Friends say that one of my strong points was the ability to converse in a rapid and analytical manner. It was always a joy to me to keep people laughing. But where is the fun in life now that this capacity has virtually disappeared from one day to the next?

Reading historian Loe de Jong's book *Struggling To My Feet* [Opkrabbelen], I recognize many of the problems he had to deal with after his brain hemorrhage. For example, he writes, '.... the region which has now been closed off has cost me not only part of my memory but part of my emotional life as well. I have become more isolated.' And later: 'I can't talk so easily. Sure, I can make a start and generally express what I want...'

I can also begin a conversation full of enthusiasm, react at full speed, banter wittily, enjoy the interaction, but my pleasure in it is also short-lived. Like a thief in the night, the pressure on my skull and face steals up on me in the course of conversation, making it impossible for me to function. The longer I try to continue in my usual fashion, the less control I have over what I say. Before I know it I have recklessly promised something, or stirred something up I didn't really want to get into. In addition, my slight stammer becomes more pronounced and I have great difficulty articulating, forcing me to slow down the pace. The sentences no longer flow, I have trouble finding the right words, until finally I get stuck and decide to stop talking.

I identify with De Jong when he says, 'It makes me tired', but that is putting it mildly. It exhausts me completely. And I have become more isolated as a result. The best proof of this is my empty calendar.

Psychologically, I am in a very weak position when I allow myself to be drawn into conversation. I lose all heart to continue, while the zest for conversation was once so ingrained in me. Wherever I used to be strong and swift I now plod along so sluggishly. Unless I want to spend the rest of the day in bed, totally shattered from talking and active listening, I must take care to steer all the stimuli descending on me each day in the right direction. But that is exactly the problem. It is no longer possible for me to actively initiate anything, yet if I want to influence the flow of stimuli, I must first analyze them in detail. There is no other way. 'Almost none of the billions of stimuli continually ˏ reaching our senses penetrate to our consciousness. And that is all for the best, since they would drive us crazy,' writes psychologist Piet Vroon in a newspaper article. But I am being driven stark raving mad by all these billions of stimuli, boring unasked into my brain in various ways. In the first place through my eyes.

A few examples. I can get dizzy even when sitting, simply by watching the people around me move. My remedy then is to sit with my back to them. I also get dizzy when I try to look around me while walking, and looking up makes it very difficult for me to keep my balance. This means that I must first stop and spread my legs wide before trying to look at anything. When I cycle, everything is fine as long as I go straight ahead, with the saddle in the lowest position. But when I have to change direction or cross an intersection I have problems.

Trying to avoid the stimuli entering via my ears also demands sophisticated strategies. Why does a phone call trigger pain in my ears? Why am I oversensitive to noise? Why do people scream like that over the phone, I'm not deaf, am I? Our telephone has a volume adjustment button, which of course is set as low as possible. So why does it always produce such a devilish racket? With some callers, the voices and even background noises are excruciating, piercing me to the bone and forcing me to stop the conversation immediately.

The only thing I can do to protect myself is to ignore the phone and shut off the bell. And when I want to make a call myself I use a hands-free phone so I don't need to bring it near my ear.

At movement therapy, with six women in a garage, there is always a lot of chatting before and after the lesson. Since the acoustics in the garage are terrible, I always sit quietly in a corner. Even when someone comes right up to me to ask how things are going, I shut myself off. I put my hands over my ears and don't answer, hoping they will stop asking about what to me seems self-evident.

And then there are the stimuli reaching my body via the sense of touch. Often, they give me the feeling that I don't fit properly in the space around me. The more people walking around nearby, the harder it is to avoid bumping into them. I bang my fingers when I try to grab the doorknob to open the door, particularly when I'm tired. When I bend down I bump my backside against whatever's behind me. My shoulders knock into the doorjambs. The automatic pilot that used to guide me has gone haywire. Even sitting down on a chair is no longer an easy task. If I am slightly distracted, I will land next to it rather than on it.

Finally the organs of smell and taste. These two senses have abandoned me completely, and that is also hard for me to deal with. I have always had a well-developed sense of smell, but now that too is denied me. And how. When I cook, there is not only the risk of forgetting the potatoes on the stove. Even when they start to burn my nose will notice nothing. No stench is foul enough to get me hurrying back to the kitchen, with all the obvious consequences.

And the burnt hunk of leather in my mouth no longer deserves the name of tongue. All tastes have vanished. My palate feels odd and prickly. All my taste buds were instantly transformed into sleeping beauties. Will they ever wake?

Only now when I no longer have them do I realize how priceless these faculties are. By enhancing the quality of life, they make you feel safe and secure, a feeling I will have to live without from now on.

Where Is My Head?

I realize that I am but a shadow of the personality I was before the traffic accident. How am I to hold onto my so cherished temperament? And what has become of my once inexhaustible energy? Has it all been run into the ground? How can I build it all up again and who can help me?

When each time you make a date with someone it leads to protracted painful complaints, you put the idea of socializing out of your head. Nonetheless, I still need to practice, but with whom and when? How long will I stay on my feet? How much time will it take me to recover after a chat and how can I make that time shorter?

Sometimes I ignore the pain and pressure and say to myself: "Come on girl, show some grit!" But that only makes the symptoms worse: my cheeks glow even more fiercely and my forehead gets hotter and hotter. When I reach that stage, and it catches me by surprise every time, I'm ready to burst into tears. Wincing and dizzy from pain, thoroughly miserable and lonely.

It is so contradictory: talking makes me feel lonely. After all, hasn't sharing joys and sorrows with others always been the most natural thing in the world? In his book *Hier en nu leven in de geest* ("Living Here and Now in the Spirit"), Henri Nouwen writes that healing always begins with the sharing of pain. But the only remedy for my pain is to completely shut myself off and do nothing, forbidding everyone to enter my room or make any kind of noise in the house.

And woe betide anyone who takes no heed of my proscriptions, for I will spring like a spider from the corner of my web and sink my fangs into my prey.

I am unbearable, that much is clear. I demand silence in my home. A proverb I often used to hear runs: "Sorrow shared is sorrow pared". I now add "except in the case of brain injury".

The tears run down my face when I read Loe de Jong's words: "...all subtlety of thought has been lost, the speed with which I used to make connections, the ease with which I could move from one domain to another within my mind. Everything has become slower, more sluggish, increasingly drained of color and grace ..." Finally, someone who not only can put my problems clearly into words but also shares them with me. I have uttered the same lament so many times, but up to now everyone around me has cheerfully replied: "You're not doing so badly!" At such moments I feel not only lonely but also totally misunderstood. When people downplay and trivialize the problem it's enough to make my hair stand on end.

De Jong's is one of the first books I read after the accident and it took me six months to get through it. It became my personal consolation, my bible. I would have liked to write to De Jong, but was incapable of executing any of the plans I conceived. By chance I had bought the book a month before my accident, because I was interested in how intelligent people experience problems, tackle them and make the best of them. After the accident, the book was ready to hand.

Brain injury is not a disease. It always has an obvious external cause: violence. An accident happens. You get whacked on the head by a roofing tile during a storm, a pile of bricks falls on you at a construction site, you tumble off a ladder while cleaning the gutter. You have to recover from the resulting injury. The characteristic feature of a brain injury is that you are brought unconscious to the nearest hospital by an ambulance, sirens wailing. You find yourself in a life-threatening situation demanding admission to intensive care and followed by treatment in the hospital neurological ward. At the present time, most brain injuries are caused by traffic accidents. Riding a bicycle or a moped, driving a car. Whether it's your own stupid fault or someone else's. It can happen to anyone.

The main difference with chronic diseases such as rheumatoid arthritis or MS is that the patient with a brain injury must travel a different route to recovery. He or she was nearly dead, but must climb as it were back out of the grave and stumble up an almost impassable mountain path to become somewhat human again. Most such patients, even under the most favorable circumstances, must learn to walk again. They must learn to keep their balance. It is as if you can't find your way in your own environment.

Some remain stuck forever in this scrambling phase. Others climb up from the depths again, not only in terms of their motor systems but cognitively as well. But always slowly. Recovery from traumatic brain injury is a very slow process. A question of years. Years of rest and isolation and endless exercise.

The process of increasing your motor skills can indeed give you a big kick, as little by little you gain more control over that recalcitrant body. But often, too, the countless limitations to which you are subject will make their presence increasingly felt as you travel the road to recovery.

The neurologist warned me that for the time being I would be capable of very little. At first I thought stubbornly: it won't be that bad. But it is that bad. I am totally incompetent.

I have to bathe in the tub because standing under the shower is too difficult. Washing my hair is an exhausting exercise and putting it in curlers is a hopeless task for my leaden arms. I can't put on pantyhose, can't bend over to tie my shoes or clip my toenails, and the time of elegant high heels is over. From now on I am condemned to flat shoes.

When getting dressed I have to sit down to put on my trousers and socks. But how do I manage to ensure that I actually sit down on the chair? Gently lower my body onto it? No, it always ends up with a jolt that reverberates in my head. Perhaps a stool would be better? But that's even harder to aim for, and once you're sitting it's much more tiring than a chair.

Going up and down stairs I raise my legs as high as I can. When I walk I swing my arms round like a windmill to keep my balance.

I can't go through a doorway without bumping into it.

The problem of bringing dishes from the sink to the cupboard has been solved with the help of a shopping basket.

Cooking is beyond me. Even when it comes to a simple recipe for sauerkraut my mind goes blank. First I have to find all the things I need, which takes an enormous amount of time. Where did I put that pan? I'm sure I have sauerkraut in stock, but where is it? And then my amazement when I finally find everything: how odd this stuff looks, is it really sauerkraut?

I am constantly disoriented or confused. In bed I have no idea where my head is. Is it lying on the pillow or the other way round? Other times I have the feeling I'm lying diagonally in bed, with my legs raised.

My senses betray me. Again and again, I surprise Willem with my strange questions, even though he always says soothingly that everything is normal.

To exercise my brain a little, I regularly consult my diary: what did I do yesterday, last week, what's on for today? I sigh with relief when no activities involving others are scheduled. The problem lies not so much in getting around; it's not just that I have a little trouble walking. The list of complaints is longer and vaguer. It is even hard to say exactly what I have trouble with.

I am constantly being caught unawares. It must be nearly impossible to live with me. I become scatterbrained when I have to organize anything, call someone up, look after money, keep track of names and addresses, travel. Looking up names and numbers in a telephone book takes hours and forces me to literally rack my brains. When I concentrate on looking for something I can feel my brains close up and stiffen into a thick porridge.

By now I have been made painfully aware of my incapacity to handle incoming phone calls.

What happens when I simply pick up the phone? My head feels like it's being given electroshock treatment. If I nonetheless persist (Be tough! Don't let it get to you!), my whole skull is soon ablaze. The pressure on my ears and head becomes unbearable. But if I don't let it get me down and just keep talking, my face and forehead begin to burn as well. My cheeks glow. At that point I come to the end of my rope and finally hang up, saying I'm on fire.

Since I am turned into a total dizzy-groggy zombie by all the unsolicited intrusions, I have asked Willem to cancel my business phone number. My family name, address and telephone number will also be deleted from the phone book. My by now ancient answering machine has vanished into my dear son's student house.

It is a real bloodletting: a piece of me is now officially dead. I am disappearing into the void, I no longer exist. My visibility and accessibility will disintegrate in no time.

It took a good deal of persuasion to convince Willem that my situation was really unbearable and that these measures had to be taken. But now that I'm over the first hurdle I am beginning to develop a taste for this way of life.

But our joint private number never stops ringing: suppliers, business contacts, concerned friends and acquaintances. Everyone intrudes into my living room with requests, appointments or "May I speak to Willem?".

This too is coming to an end. When I'm asked to pass on messages, I forget them immediately. Notes get lost, numbers are not taken down correctly or vanish in piles of paper. Willem is cross: "You can still take a message, can't you?" Well, yes, I can, provided it's a single message, and that I repeat it to myself and immediately jot down the name of the caller. But that takes an unspeakable amount of effort, all that listening, writing, answering. The only thing I can really count on is a red-hot splitting headache each time I do it.

When Willem answers the phone himself he is often ruthlessly honest: 'Yes, sure, she's here, just let me call her.' To make it clear to him and our student sons that the situation is really serious, I insist that they no longer give out our number and address to third parties. Not to clients or colleagues, and no listings in yearbooks either.

This is easier said than done. Because I am no longer willing to be browbeaten by every Tom, Dick and Harry, all telephone bells in the house are shut off (despite some heavy sputtering at first).

Perhaps it seems that I am now browbeating my home environment, but closer observation may lead to a more balanced view of the situation. A home office is always a source of considerable commotion. Many doctor's wives nowadays also insist that the office be far from the home, and they don't suffer from brain injury.

Since my radical decision, our telephones only indicate a caller on the line by means of flickering red lights. What bliss, what peace! Finally I can take care of a simple chore at home without having to launch into ten other things that I won't finish properly anyway.

The frequent flickering of the lights makes it clear how necessary this action was. Only in the bedroom does the telephone still wake me up sometimes. Here the solution is to stuff the thing under the bed or a pillow. Time and time again, irritated and overwrought, I threaten to rip the phone out of the wall or throw it out the window. "Leave me in peace, for heaven's sake!"

Meanwhile I discover that my driving license is about to expire. The way things stand, the idea of having to take a driving test again scares the daylights out of me.

My bruised head will never be able to grasp the theory and driving on the freeway is also a thing of the past.

Four months after the accident I drove ("You can do it, Mom. There's a first time for everything.", said my oldest son) to the station in our home town for the first time. I came home dead tired after this tremendous three-mile journey. I decided at the last moment to take the straight main road rather than the winding village lanes but it was still an enormous task. Although I had been an expert driver since the age of eighteen, I crept behind the wheel like a mouse and could barely bring myself to push the speedometer up to 30.

Now what? Luckily the family doctor had already asked encouragingly: "Are you starting to drive a little again?". So he and the neurologist see no problem in it. But why can't I glide smoothly round the curves? Why do I get so tired from all those vehicles swarming around me?

I decide to ask for an extension. I kept copies of my previous application to make it easier to fill in the forms next time, but now that I need them I can't find them anywhere. I search till I'm ready to collapse and feel totally desperate. In tears I ask Willem to take care of it for me. His only reaction is: "You can handle that yourself, can't you?"

"No way", I tell him, fuming.

Willem frowns with irritation. In the end, the paperwork is obtained for me, with a little yellow sticker on the form to show me where to put my signature. As if I was illiterate. Which I practically am. All the lines dance before my eyes. I look like a moron.

My passport also appears to have expired. That means I need to have passport photos made. And this too takes all my energy for a whole day. I drive downtown at ten in the morning so that I can easily find a place to park. The photographer plants me on a stool and says, "Sit still". But I can't manage it. He gives me a chair.

Afterwards I curiously examine the result. Sure enough, a glassy look as if I am not of this world. A wax museum head with a smile forced on a painful mouth.

Is that strange person me? In my new passport I am suddenly an inch shorter than I really am, and that's how I feel too: cut down to size.

Time after time I put articles and books I want to read aside, thinking "I can't manage this now, but later…'. After a year, the door of the smallest study in the house (five square meters), where the boxes containing my backlog of reading matter are stored, can no longer be shut. The room opens onto the entrance hall, so if something is not done about this pigsty soon it will be impossible to open the front door too.

The size of my little retreat never bothered me before. By nature I am an orderly and conscientious person. Moreover, it also had advantages. Since it could accommodate only one person at a time, I was never bothered by uninvited chitchat. Anyone who did come in soon fell prey to claustrophobia ("How do you stand it in here?") and got out in a hurry. There was no need for cold stares.

Another advantage of my private world was the large window overlooking a bird-filled bramble patch. Whenever my thoughts wandered off I could gaze at this natural aviary and admire the pairs of goldfinches and hawfinches feasting on the berries.

But these days I no longer get much work done. I have had to cancel all my subscriptions and memberships in various professional organizations.. Canceling them was a bloodletting and a turning point, but it was also perhaps a weight off my mind. Had I clung too long to the idea that my problems would one day be over? Had I been too optimistic? Should I have focused all my attention on looking for things I could still do rather than dwelling on what I could not yet or no longer do?

Before my accident I read three national newspapers each day, now I don't even read one. The discovery that I can no longer read swiftly, running my eyes diagonally down the page, is a shock. There is nothing wrong with my vision, but reading makes me dizzy. Also after reading a couple of words I lose track of the line and can't find it again.

I must thus develop a strategy to boost my reading capacity. All the letters dance before my eyes. I need to use a ruler. To begin with, I look for easy reading. Short pieces. Glossy women's magazines make an appearance in our house. But initially even leafing through these magazines gives me a headache.

I start saving the science supplements in the newspaper and set myself the task of reading one or two articles each week. I can only manage it with the help of a ruler and a highlighter. I keep relevant cuttings about the brain or related topics in a box, whether or not I read them. I prefer articles in large type.

Reading books is even more troublesome. I start by looking up words that interest me in the index and then read only the paragraph referred to. But even that sounds easier that it is. Using the index is itself a problem. But I persevere, armed with my highlighter. At least I manage to obtain information this way, even if there is as yet no question of making connections between the things I read.

I put yellow stickers on pages that interest me. But since I don't write any notes on them, I end up later with a book full of little stickers without knowing why I put them there.

One day, when I don't have to cook or do any other chores, I decide to read a whole book. And what a book! Big letters, simple plot, few characters: the story of a couple and their children who buy and renovate a country house in France. Traditional and sweet. It keeps me happy for hours.

To practice writing I take a bright blue notebook and copy out the sayings and proverbs I find in newspaper obituaries. They are the first notices I can manage to read again. Short and digestible, yet they make sense. It suits my somber mood.

During a short stay with Willem in a hotel with a swimming pool two years after the accident, I swim again for the first time. I swim, albeit with arms that feel like flabby paddles. My breaststroke is sluggish and stiff. I can also manage to float on my back. And so there I float, the once fervent swimmer of lap after lap!

Now for the backstroke. But as soon as I try it, I get the feeling that my head is already about to hit the wall. I turn around in alarm. Still a long way to go. This happens over and over. My automatic pilot lets me down again and again. I can no longer navigate with the 'eyes in the back of my head'.

Since this also happens if I have to step backwards when walking, it doesn't really worry me. On the contrary, recognizing the same spatial problem stimulates me to do something about it. It is something I will have to practice.

I am walking more and more now. One walk in Holland, on the dike between the built-up fields, I still remember very well.

It is a clear day with a stiff breeze. I am easily thrown off balance and with my jerky walk have great difficulty on the unpaved road. The process control mechanism in my brain is definitely on the blink. I keep my eyes on the ground.

I have to stand still when I want to look at the scenery around me. Pain in my neck and pressure on my head.

Absolute concentration, as if I was climbing in the Himalayas.

I am not the only walker, I now notice. Judging by my zigzag walk, they must think I've been hitting the sherry pretty early today—and I don't even like to drink.

I still have to get used to my faltering, protesting body.

Under these circumstances I can hardly think. If I glance to the side I am sure to fall over. I must stand still before I can turn my head.

My movements are anything but flowing.

I walk in the soft alpine snow. Each time I sink into it, I have great difficulty recovering my balance. The worst thing is that the speed of the movement gives me a pain in the head. I can't describe how that feels: disoriented, acute headache, jolts in my neck.

I feel terribly disabled, ask myself what I'm doing here on this rough terrain. Torturing myself? It makes me deeply unhappy. Words fail me and I burst into tears, startling Willem and the children.

If I can't even do this any longer, does it mean I should never go to the mountains again? I can't bear the thought. I'm not yet ready to give it up. I'll just have to restrict my movements, make sure I choose the easiest paths.

I love the Alps so much, get so much joy out of walking there. Must it all now come to an end?

An Exercise in Pain

For the first year and a half after the accident, I had a tremendous amount of pain. I was unable to clean the kitchen sink and draining board, or even grate nutmeg. Washing and combing my hair gave me pain, as did every movement of my face. Even nodding or blinking were best avoided.

After every eye operation I was forbidden to wash my hair myself for at least six weeks. Initially, I could think of nothing better than to dutifully go to the hairdresser, bandaged eye and all. My vanity, however, obliged me to do so at least twice a week. A total of twenty-four appointments, while previously I had gone at most nine times a year. Leaving my hair unwashed was not an option. I simply had to put up with this new torment.

What caused all this pain? In the first place the position of my neck, leaning backwards over the washbasin. Secondly by my head being handled and massaged. 'Don't touch me there, please use cold water, set the blow-drier on cold. Don't shake my head!'. Remedy: earplugs in, washbasin set as high as possible (obliging the beautician to stand on a stool), only wash once instead of twice, don't talk.

I usually asked the hairdresser to use cold water. This was often impossible. The temperature is the same for everyone, but it is much too hot for a contusio cerebri patient. If the hairdresser started right in without waiting for the water to warm up it was better for me. Then in any case I had a cold start.

The first thing I always had to do at the hairdresser's was find a quiet out-of-the-way spot where I would not be blinded by all the mirrors and could sit as far as possible from the chatter of the other clients and the music, which irritated me even through my earplugs.

In the spring, three and a half years after the accident, I manage to make all these arrangements myself for the first time. Over the telephone I try to make an appointment with a beautician I know who can make hair-washing into a relatively pleasurable experience (in so far as this is possible when I have to lean over backwards). She has subtly rotating fingers that can softly massage the skin of my head. For if I get just anyone to wash my hair, then I am at the mercy of the gods! I have to be handled with velvet gloves.

But despite my preparations I am given a rather coarse wash that again degenerates into a headache. The skin of my head is transformed into a sensitive hard-ribbed washboard. The result: pain, pain, pain.

Slowly, supporting myself as best I can, I make my way through the beauty parlor to the till, where I pay in cash.

I look back on my earlier experiences with pain. As a toddler of three, my hair in pigtails, in my little smock and matching panties, with my little hand in father's big one, I climb trustfully into a taxi to go to a surgeon who will cut away the hairy birthmark on my thigh. In those days, all potential sources of cancer had to be removed. I still remember the taxi ride as an adventure, but not climbing up onto the surgeon's table. Now that I was there, no escape was possible. I must have sobbed and protested considerably, but to no avail. There was nothing my dear father could do to save me, although the fact that he could stay in the room gave me some comfort, eased my little heart.

The surgeon makes a joke about a slice of gingerbread when he shows me the cut-off strip of flesh. There was a lot of iodine and blood, and I had eighteen stitches. The nurse wraps me in layer after layer of bandages, so that I look like a mummy by the time I'm ready to go home, rather more subdued than I was on the way there.

The pain begins when the anesthetic wears off, but it doesn't last long. And I heal quickly.

Another memory dates from the age of seven when my eye had just been operated on to correct my congenital cataract and squint. I was treated in two stages at the *Ooglijdersgasthuis* ('Eye Patients Hospital') in Utrecht. The first time I don't shed a tear, although I am conscious the whole time. The second time there are complications once I return home. I am racked with pain in the eye that has been operated on and take to my bed, covering the eye with my hand. The upshot is that I must immediately return to Utrecht, where I get injections into my ailing eye. While mother and the eye doctor try to calm me down, I scream and thrash about. The needle seems as huge as a fly sprayer. I screech my head off.

I don't know any more how many nurses it took to hold me down, but the doctor was called Jansen and had a mop of curly hair.

The infection was quickly over, helped by disinfectant eye drops. And the pain did not come back.

A third memory of pain goes back to shortly after my fortieth birthday. My bad eye, blinded by cataract, began to act strangely: it throbbed, it turned bright red and shed tears, it felt like it was being sucked through a straw, then suddenly floated free again. When I bent over all these symptoms worsened and it felt like a rock-hard marble.

Once again I am a true eye patient and rush to the Eye Patients Hospital. The head of the clinic comes by and I hear words like glaucoma and enucleation. This last word I recall is an archaic term for 'explain' or 'disclose'. 'What is to be disclosed?' I wonder. I want to know what's being cooked up behind my back but before I know it a young doctor has taken me by the arm and we are standing in front of the nurse in admissions. Slowly the realization dawns: they're going to operate. Since I first want to consider the options at home, I struggle free. I say that I want to get an idea of what's going on before anything is removed.

Despite the atropine the eye is still sickly. The miserable thing keeps giving me pain. So back I go. This time Prof. Winkelman discovers that there is still some response from my nearly blind glaucomatous eye. He decides on a minor operation that for the time being will allow me to keep this 'quite ugly eye'.

The head of the clinic gives me a mini-seminar on glaucoma. Amazed and interested I follow his explanation of the minor operation intended to reduce the pressure on my eyeball. Ultimately, Winkelman drills four little holes to allow the watery fluid within the eyeball to circulate freely through the chambers of the eye again, which reduces the eye pressure to normal proportions.

It takes awhile for the pain to disappear, but then I am free of complaints. Until a couple of years later when I can no longer lie down or sleep, vomit repeatedly at night and have pain on one side of my head. The symptoms return without warning sometimes three times a day and in the middle of one such attack I go to the University Hospital. There the diagnosis is acute glaucoma. In the case of a blind eye that means 'enucleation'. If something offends you, tear it out, it says in the Bible somewhere. The time for this has now come.

I come round from the anesthetic in the recovery room, hear the beeps of a heart monitor and murmuring around me. A voice asks: 'Are you awake already?' I can see nothing, which is very distressing. I become aware of a tremendous pain in my eye. With great difficulty I keep myself from screaming, I have never felt pain like this. It feels like a red-hot poker is stuck in my eye socket. From the frying pan into the fire, the pain is much worse than before the operation.

Willem sits next to me while a nurse gives me morphine to ease the pain. The nurse has already cautiously told me that the implant I am getting will make the pain somewhat worse. 'No pain, no gain', the saying goes, and it couldn't be truer in my case. My eye socket feels like a razor blade has been stuck in it. Each time I try to focus my eye on something, the pain shoots through my eye socket. For fourteen long days I have to bear this piercing pain.

I can't stand pity. I won't easily let myself be pushed into the 'poor soul' routine. At an early age I developed a defensive toughness, saying 'Oh, it wasn't so bad. I thought it would be *much* worse!', drawing out that 'much' as long as possible for emphasis. As a result, I was soon regarded as a 'tough cookie' when with knocking knees I had to climb up on the operating table for the umpteenth time.

Neither surgeons nor nurses have any time for crybabies. When I was complimented on being a 'tough cookie' it helped me to keep my courage up too.

Even after my accident I still like to be complimented on lying so calmly on the operating table. I am very susceptible to such praise and it motivates me to keep up my stoic attitude by thinking of pleasant things that have brought me joy. I almost feel it as a rude interruption of my reflections when the surgeon says that all has gone well and the operation is nearly over.

During the first re-suturing of the implant this attitude works fine. The eye surgeon warns me when I might feel something, for example when he pulls the sutures tight, but that is not really painful. And when he injects the anesthetic he says that it might hurt. It does, three times in a row. Before my brain injury I might well have asked why it hurts, but by now I have taught myself to think: let it be, a person can't know and control everything.

Initially the hunt for the nasty tormentors in my jaw and mouth produces no results. Until finally a new abscess reveals the long-sought spot where this devil is hiding. The dental surgeon speedily removes the broken root (apex resection) and stitches it all neatly up again. Somewhat uprooted but mainly unburdened I leave the University Hospital. Is this fiendish demon now banished for good?

These experiences with pain have taught me that there are two types of pain, acute and chronic. If I had to choose, then I would pick acute pain as the lesser of the two evils. Acute pain has a more or less fixed duration, its contours can be grasped, it can be fought. You can reduce this pain to a bearable level. But once some hooligan has knocked you flat you will soon be suffering chronic pain. And then what? Never before in my life had I been troubled by headaches. That was a blessing. It had been my fortune to have a good, clear head until a moped torpedoed my body.

By now I have received the most diverse advice in response to my complaints about pain: take drugs, go to the pain clinic, try acupuncture, see a neurologist, go to a different hospital for a second opinion, take a nice vacation, spoil yourself in a hotel, have your hair done, go to a beauty parlor. And then more often than not I was asked whether I might not just be suffering from menopause. To that question I can now answer from experience 'no, that was not yet a problem'. Those little vicissitudes started only seven years after the accident.

As always, of course, my brain injury makes it difficult for me to make a sensible choice based on all that well-intended advice. Meanwhile I am developing into a chronic complainer. I suffer, as I make sure everyone knows, from pressure on my skull, ears, cheeks, cheekbones, front and back teeth, back, neck and nose and my head feels like someone is constantly pulling my hair.

But my nervous system is really in bad shape and no matter how I address it ('You have nothing to say, I'm the boss here') it has absolutely no effect.

There are of course all sorts of painkillers available. I have been given three, each one stronger than the last. First paracetamol, of which I never took more than six tablets a day after the hospital, while the maximum daily dose is eight to ten. If paracetamol doesn't do the trick, the narcotic codeine is given. Then comes morphine, in the form of suppository, drink or tablet, with the morphine injection as a last resort.

Once out of the hospital I very much wanted to cut down on the high doses of paracetamol I was using. The family doctor, who visited me weekly, was in complete agreement.

I had two reasons for wanting to reduce my drug intake. In the first place, those things have not been made to improve your health. 'Prolonged and frequent use of paracetamol is not advisable', warns the manufacturer in a brochure in the family doctor's waiting room. If you take more than the prescribed daily dose you're asking for liver problems. Secondly, I hoped as soon as possible to regain some control over where and when I had pain and how bad the pain could be.

I want to get to the bottom of my complaints and pinpoint them.

Balancing on the Beam

Four years after the accident, I make a list for myself of its continuing effects on me.

- After an hour writing or talking I feel intense pressure on my head, eye, jaws, ears and forehead.
- I still leave the room when the children come home full of stories about their doings.
- I still don't go out in the evenings, i.e. no theater, opera, chamber music or visits to children or friends.
- In the weekends I sometimes see intimate friends, for no more than an hour, preferably a couple, with Willem there to take the lead so that I can lie low.
- I never feel free to speak my mind, and if I do it makes me dizzy, groggy, dead tired.
- If I exceed my limits I suffer blazing heat in my head and can't sleep.
- I need a ridiculous amount of sleep, ten hours a night on average.
- I must prepare myself thoroughly, in complete isolation, in order to calm down enough to be able to sleep.
- I prefer to do things alone, because company takes too much energy.
- Listening to music is no longer one of my pastimes.
- I no longer receive unexpected visitors.
- I don't answer the telephone.
- Sports? Sometimes a little golf, maximum nine holes, while I previously used to play in competitions with great enthusiasm.
- Crossing the street without tottering and wobbling is a big problem.

- Travelling on my own is much too complicated: too many stimuli and choices.
- I only drive the car on familiar terrain, in a radius of 10 miles around our house.
- Walking and talking divides my attention and makes me stumble.
- Above all, I must not try to combine things, doing one thing at a time is hard enough.

Before the accident I went to Anaheim, California for a scholarly conference. In my free time I visited a sort of panoramic movie theatre in Disneyland. The film I saw in this circular theatre was of a great ship plunging through an enormous storm.

Along with many others, I stood between barriers looking at the screen. And each time the ship yawed through the sea we clutched the so-called rail to keep from falling. We were laughing, screaming, howling. Our visual perceptions influenced our sense of balance. What we saw caused our brains to produce stimuli affecting our equilibrium, which could not adjust fast enough so that we staggered even though the floor beneath our feet was not moving.

On television I watch ten-year-old girls scooting over the balance beam, now and then making mighty leaps. When one of them falls off the beam the commentator says 'Before the jump she threw back her head and that causes problems with balance', adding a bit later 'She is very concentrated, keeping her eyes on the beam'.

It reminds me of my own situation. How often have I tried to explain that it is as if I am walking on a balance beam and must keep my eyes focused on the ground? These girls don't try to talk while performing their feats, do they? If they do they will fall, just like me. Can they look to the side while balancing on the beam? How long can they keep up their balancing acts? And how many hours a week do they have to train for it?

Dizziness can take various forms. When the neurologist asks me an apparently simple question ('Are you dizzy?'), I will probably answer in the negative. Because sitting across from him in a chair with my back supported I really am not dizzy. But after my accident I find it hard to distinguish the circumstances in which I do get dizzy.

A patient with traumatic brain injury is incapable, certainly for the first two years, of unraveling complicated concepts. Let alone critically evaluating his or her own situation. And definitely not an abstract concept like dizziness, a generic term for a wide range of sensations and a slightly vertiginous feeling in the head.

But when I do get dizzy there must be such a weird look in my eyes, for everyone rushes to offer help. This one brings me a chair, that one calls out 'Do you feel unwell?', most of them take me resolutely by the arm and lead me away. That unsteadiness of mine evokes pity. Although I always say I'm not going to fall, most people won't leave it at that and extend a helping hand. Then I usually have poor control over my legs, which exacerbates the clumsy motor system. On top of that I always squeeze my eyes shut to make my way through the swarm of people, enormous obstacles for me. But if people suddenly move I bump right into them. And when I try to form proper sentences to indicate what I want and where, they deteriorate into stutter and stammer. My internal coordination is a mess.

As soon as I am in a quiet room with one other person, I can talk and walk again and act somewhat more normally. My poor head feels like a magnetic field being drawn by a magnet to a single point. Heavy pressure on head and ears. It drives me up the wall.

After my accident, I could still read the headline in the newspaper without a ruler: 'Drugs for dizziness almost always useless'. But now I can read the article too. One of the conclusions is as follows: 'Not only is dizziness not an illness, it is not even a symptom. It is rather an umbrella term used by patients for the most diverse forms of unsteadiness.'

Dizziness usually has to do with our sense of balance. This sense is influenced by at least three regulatory systems in our body and the cause of dizziness may be found in each of these: the inner ear, the central nervous system and the eyes and the senses that register depth perception in our muscles and joints.

The remedy for this type of syndrome is often a balanced lifestyle. Complaints such as headache, neck and back pain, high blood pressure, heartburn and insomnia can also be alleviated by taking things a bit easier, giving sufficient time and attention to sports and exercise, and making provision for relaxation and recreation. Many people complaining of dizziness are not really sick but chronically overburdened.

Three years after the accident I went cross-country skiing for the first time. It was April, late in the season. One day I set off, for the second time that week. Willem and the boys had left very early, wanting to ski on the glacier for a change. I was happily on my own. Although I was already in bed by nine the night before, I was still a late riser. It was ten o'clock that morning before I had washed and groomed myself at my own pace.

I didn't dare climb the steep snow path to the public road with slippery flat shoes. First I had to dig five steps in the snow, a staggering task. New snow is heavy, that much I knew. By the time I had to come back, I would have absolutely no energy left. My men weren't bothered by it at all, they just stomped through the deep snow on their long Dutch legs. So then I left, supported by two ski poles, rucksack on my back, in climbing boots with crampons, to Xavier's chalet next to the ski run. I sat on a bench in his front garden, with a view of a four-thousand-meter peak, to change my footwear. My skis were hanging under the balcony on the side of the house. I left my rucksack behind. I made my way to the children's piste, somewhat further than the 'adult piste', and hung my body warmer on the post marking the start of the run. Fortunately there was no one around. Why did I pick the children's piste? Because it was tiny, with hardly any slope, and thus seemed to be a feasible goal. Start with one round and work up to three or more? Should be possible! But there was something wrong with the snow. Too much sun, so that my skis stuck and braked like mad things, while last time they had glided so smoothly. Jerking and bumping along, first faster, then slower, my neck and head soon felt like they were being whipped. So much pain was not the idea. Above all that unexpected braking, caused by spots of mushy snow, soon made it necessary to give the whole thing up. Dizzy and with my head on fire, I walked back. And was nearly knocked off my feet by a cross-country skier, who came whooshing down from the top of the hill at breakneck speed right in front of me. His yell spared me a new accident. How could that happen? I had stopped and looked carefully, I thought. This was a new dent in my self-confidence. I had seen him with my own eyes at the top of the hill, looking around to see if the coast was clear. Did I think I had just enough time to cross in front of him? No, next to the adult piste was a speed skater's course and a footpath and I had mixed them up. My powers of spatial perception abandoned me when I was dizzy. While this was a traffic-free village I had been familiar with for years. In Holland I would not go out on the roads with such a dizzy head. I would feel a loss of control, as had now been confirmed. I should have waited even longer, until there was really no one in sight, before crossing those three paths. I was upset by the dismal start to the day: completely worn out, nothing to show for it, and a near-accident. My mood dropped below zero.

But three years later I put on skis again: on the baby slope. Maarten has skied to a hotel with my skis, while I walk there in my climbing boots, ski boots in my rucksack, leaning on two ski poles.

And there I go. First I follow him down, a strange giddy feeling, but I want to keep going, so then I do it alone. I am given a few technical tips: edge the lower ski, keep your knees in, keep your weight in front by leaning forward in your boots and hold your ski poles in front of your body, not next to it. Maarten thinks my skis are not so good for edging, and a little short besides.

Three times with the children's lift, then I stay up there and move on to the hotel, where I change boots on the terrace. I leave my skis in the rack for tomorrow, when I intend to do it again without help. Another milestone!

Walking on skis or climbing does give me pain in my neck and head, a bumpy feeling, very tiring. And my forehead is overheated.

Since I can ski slowly, using two ski poles, I can avoid the kids. Looking quickly to the side is not an option. The dizzy feeling is not so bad but I do sweat heavily.

Like a true gladiator, Maarten clears the piste for me. All this watching out for his mother leaves him terribly weary.

When people see me doing things again in the years following my accident, they often think: "How nice that she's able to travel again—or play tennis or golf, or go skiing or shopping…" How many of them realize that such instances are often one-off events, or that I will have to pay for my efforts with three sleepless nights, exhaustion and pain?

In the summer I once again take short walks in the mountains, preferably on broad, paved paths. If I attempt narrow little tracks or steep inclines I'm asking for trouble, despite my walking stick. Although my condition has clearly improved, I am still plagued by neck and back pains. Not to mention the fact that my thighs and calves ache all day long, but that was to be expected.

On August 15 there is a chapel festival in our mountain village, with an outdoor mass and music in the meadow in front of the little church. It begins at ten in the morning, a good time for me since I can easily make it without hurrying. I bring along the aluminum folding chair Willem gave me for my birthday so that I don't have to wobble on my feet for an hour.

The sounds of the band and the choir waft out over the snowy mountaintops. In any case, they are not drilling into my ears. The clanging of cowbells in the distance mingles with the voice of the priest.

After the service comes the "apero". The local hotelkeeper and his son keep the glasses full. Xavier and his daughter Carmen see to it that my glass is topped up with juice. Carmen sits next to me for a friendly chat and tells me about her trip to Sienna. I see other people I know and since I am in no shape to hobble over to them they come to me.

So there I sit, welded to the spot. If I want to look at someone, I must first bend my head backwards as far as I can.

To my distress the drums of the band begin to roll. Even outdoors I can't bear that sound, let alone keep chatting away like the others. I don't feel like putting my earplugs in so I tell Carmen I'm going to call it a day. I fold up my chair and totter off homewards.

After an hour and a half at home enjoying the view, I take two golf clubs and go to the driving range to relax and hit a few balls. The last thing I want to do is talk. On the way I run into acquaintances and tell them bluntly that I want to keep walking and won't stop to chat. I couldn't care less whether they understand or not, for me it is a question of survival.

Back in the Netherlands I sometimes overreach myself and take on more than I can handle, despite all my good intentions. Last night I slept well and got up at 8.30 so that I don't need to hurry to get ready to welcome my new housekeeper at 10. I don't sit down and drink coffee with her because I want to save all my time and energy for writing.

But then I still get disturbed, by a friend who has always been there for me. The situation is most disconcerting. How am I supposed to tell her that her visit is badly timed? I can't do it. I must make it more clear to the gatekeepers who protect me from the outside world that from now on I am not to be disturbed when I'm writing.

In the afternoon I play a little tennis on the outdoor court. There are only two of us instead of the usual six, so there is more exchange of information, more return balls, and so more walking, more picking up balls, more coordination demanded of me. Without being asked, my forehead and cheeks fire up again and start to glow. Despite two breaks, I am very dizzy when it is finally over.

I prepared this evening's dinner the day before, so all I have to do is pop it in the microwave. When Willem comes home at 8 o'clock we eat and then go out for some fresh air in the nearby park. That's something I really like to do, since the rest of the day he leads a sedentary existence.

So get a move on, and lace up your hiking boots.

While the weekdays are always tiring for me, the weekends take the cake. For then I must constantly make choices, give no for an answer, when all I really want to do is simply spend time with my husband and my two student sons. There is so much to discuss.

Well before dinnertime this Saturday, things start to go wrong. I'm cooking, preparing various dishes, while trying at the same time to listen to my son, who has important things to tell me. It is impossible. I ask him to go away, to be quiet, because all that information is making me dizzy and driving me mad. I can no longer concentrate.

With a great deal of willpower, I then manage to finish cooking. But serving is too much for me, I have to leave it to the men. One of my sons takes the initiative to set the table.

They find the food delicious. Thank goodness for that, I certainly did my best. I eat little myself, the buzz of conversation overwhelms me.

I skip dessert and go off to bed.

Before I go to bed, Willem gives me a hug. Does he understand a little, comparing today with other days? During the week, when there's just the two of us, I can still take a walk in the evening, have a little chat. Not that I don't have complaints, but I can put up with them. In any case, I don't need to go to bed at 7 o'clock.

Sunday. I wake up at 8.15 in an empty house, deliciously quiet. Thanks to my excellent earplugs, I didn't even hear the men get up at 7 to start their eighteen holes.

After my breakfast of yogurt I have to almost forcibly restrain myself from rushing off to our parish church where a mass according to the Byzantine rites is being held. The idea of missing the Byzantine choir led by the young choirmaster makes me heartsick. But the crowd, the chaotic traffic, the passionate music, the greeting of acquaintances, it would all be too much for me.

My heart cries out in silence. I simply can't be pleased with my sensible decisions. Will I ever get used to being sidelined?

On Christmas Eve Willem and I walk with our rucksacks to the little supermarket in the mountain village. Naturally, it's full to bursting, as I had predicted. I write down what we need on a slip of paper and Willem squeezes inside on his own.

I find a quiet spot in the sun and sit down on the sled we have brought along. Not surprisingly, it takes him quite a while, but there is a marvelous view of the snowy four-thousand-meter peaks surrounding the valley and I don't mind the wait at all.

Suddenly an acquaintance starts talking to me. And then I hear the Frequently Asked Question: "Aren't you bitter about what happened to you?"

I realize I have never seen what good that would do. Bitterness would only have a poisonous effect. Since I am not made of stone, I have begun to express my vexations and feelings of injustice in writing. But I am doing my best to keep it from turning into a lament. It should also be good for a laugh now and then, no matter how little there is to laugh about.

I explain that my principal handicap is social amputation. And while I am saying this I'm thinking, "if that was only all there was to it!"

I ask her to stop talking about it, because I'm about to burst into tears. "There's already a lump in my throat."

Shocked, she asks: "Would you like me to go? Or will you tell me yourself when you've had enough?"

It is a big problem, for I am actually enjoying our chat. Naturally I have the nerve to cut off the conversation myself and make my way home, sled and all. But then Willem would wonder where I was.

She leaves to join our husbands, who by now are standing chatting a short distance away. Her husband comes over to say hello, but now I'm on the defensive. I just can't take it any more.

The three of them keep talking for a while on their own. Then Willem joins me and announces enthusiastically that we're invited to their place for coffee.

I don't react. What I'm thinking is: "Just leave me in peace, remember my poor aching head."

Letter to my Perpetrator

The young man who banged me into the hospital wrote this letter to Willem the following day:

> *Dear Mr. Vrakking,*
> *First of all, I want to say how truly sorry I am for all the hardship and suffering I have caused your family, especially your wife.*
> *I am writing in connection with the telephone conversation I had with your son, in which we agreed that I would send the claim form to you. I have now called the insurance company, and they told me to send the claim form to them. The insurance company will then contact both you and your insurer.*
> *I hope you will be able to forgive me, so that I can get over my weird feelings about this. Wishing your wife and family good luck and all the best,*
> *Yours truly,*
> *F.H.*

Four years later, I decide to write a letter back.

> Dear Traffic Offender and Perpetrator,
> You may be shocked by this salutation, but I prefer to call a spade a spade when there is good reason to do so. And there certainly is in this case.
> First the positive things: your letter.
> As you may know, following my accident I was admitted in an unconscious condition to the

neurological ##high-dependency ward in the University Hospital.

Even after a number of days, the reason for my admission had still not sunk in. It was a complete mystery to me. Again and again, my husband and children told me I had had a traffic accident, but it just wouldn't penetrate, and if it did I would forget it a second later.

The only thing my wounded brain could imagine was that someone had tried to murder me. When my husband told me you had written him a letter I asked him to bring it to the hospital. He didn't think that was such a good idea at first, but nonetheless a few days later your letter was tacked to my bulletin board.

Reading the letter itself was not such an easy task. All the letters were dancing a little jig before my eyes. So your letter was read aloud to me. It had no effect, I felt nothing, it was very remote from me.

What everyone automatically expected failed to happen: no feelings of hatred welled up in me, there were no feelings at all. At the very least, it seemed only proper that you let us hear from you. If you had sent a basket of fruit or flowers I probably would have been unable to bear having them near me. I think that sort of thing more appropriate for a broken leg than diffuse brain injury. (Although my family and I were still unaware that this was the case!)

For the same reason, I would have indignantly declined a visit from you to the hospital. So you did very well to take no further initiatives in that direction.

Now a few more words about how useful your letter was to me and why I actually thought it a good thing to do. It helped me enormously to realize that I had landed in the hospital because of a traffic violation committed by you. Yes, it sounds a bit strange, but my brain was injured, and I only became aware of the seriousness of this injury many months later. But the tangible evidence of the cause was now hanging on the bulletin board, so I simply had to believe it.

Whenever I regained consciousness for awhile, I looked at the wall covered with cards, telegrams and letters, including your letter, and this allowed my damaged brain to absorb new information. In any case, that much I could do.

The true cause of my involuntary stay in the hospital was you. So that mystery was solved.

When visitors came and I was unable to answer all their questions (How did it happen? Where did it happen? Aren't you furious with that moped rider?), I would point to the bulletin board as a source of information. So your letter came in handy.

What else was positive about it? The fact that you were insured when you rode around on your moped, a minimum requirement in our country. Thus really quite normal. But I want to mention it here as a positive point, since it is often not the case. A pat on the back for you and your parents.

Anyway, most of your letter was about claim forms and insurance, something I have not been involved with to this very day. Too complicated for my injured brain. And above all too emotional.

You write to my husband that you are truly sorry 'for all the hardship and suffering I have caused your family, especially your wife'. That hardship and suffering are not slight.

You have robbed me of my health. I can never work again. The many sports I used to enjoy are impossible for me now, just like most of my hobbies. Socially I no longer count, for talking and listening have become the most strenuous tasks, triggering particularly troublesome neurological complaints that only vanish with prolonged rest, which means isolating myself even from my family. So I live according to my new motto: seek silence and avoid company.

Yet I don't hate you, although I think I have every reason to. Because, with what brain I have left, I can still understand that hatred only produces negative feelings, and I know that this is not very effective if you have always had a positive attitude towards life and want to keep it that way.

Naturally, I still don't think I would jump for joy at the idea of meeting you. Anyway, I can't jump at all any more. So be warned: keep out of my way, especially with that moped of yours.

Apart from all the joy of life you have robbed me of, you have also given me something: permanent pain in my head and face. That's why I almost always refer to you as that traffic offender or that perpetrator who caused me all this grief for the sole reason that you got such a fantastic kick out of speeding, hogging the whole road in the process, even the side that was mine by right, with all the disastrous consequences I have listed above.

'I hope you will be able to forgive me, so that I can get over my weird feelings', you write to my husband. By now of course I know very well what feelings your behavior aroused and still arouses in my husband and my two sons.

Forgiveness is a big word. The consequences are too drastic for it here. Forgiveness has to do with pardoning guilt. If you steal from someone, take or borrow something without permission, you have betrayed his trust, but you can get a new chance by showing that you won't display such unwelcome behavior again. The trust between you can then be reestablished.

If you cause an accident with permanent (brain) injury, you should understand that things are slightly different.

You prefer to avoid the word 'guilt' by talking about 'weird feelings'. But your feelings are not weird at all: it is perfectly normal for you to feel guilty. *I* wasn't driving much to fast, *I* wasn't hogging your side of the road, *I* didn't knock you into the hospital. Well then!

I think it very possible for you to transform this negative guilt feeling into something positive by changing the way you drive. If you keep on with the same old driving behavior you will no doubt claim more victims. But you can do something about that yourself.

If you are interested in my new lifestyle and the many problems I have had because of you, I advise you and your fellow moped riders to sit down quietly and read the book I am writing. Perhaps then you will be less likely to shrug things like this off and you may acquire more insight into your driving habits, where one person's recklessness leads to depriving another person of much of the joy of life. My inevitable limitations affect me in the first place, of course, but they also take their toll on my husband and children.

You close your letter with the words: 'Wishing your wife and family good luck and all the best'.
I would like to end my letter by wishing you good luck in ridding yourself of those 'weird (guilt) feelings'. Above all, work hard on breaking your antisocial driving habits.
If you make the same mistake again, and whether or not you do is entirely up to you, then more people will definitely fall victim to your driving style. And you certainly don't want that, do you?
Good luck!
Sincerely,
Mrs. A. M. A. Willemsen

I decide against sending the letter.

Instead, I try once again to put myself in the perpetrator's place and write the following piece:

Conscious and Unconscious

You approach a curve at high speed, hearing and seeing nothing. You know the curve well, for you often take this road on your way from your parents' house to your own home. You are 21 years old, and fully capable of considering your driving habits as an adult.

You wear a fully closed helmet around your brain (your most prized possession, after all) to keep you safe from cars. You hear nothing, no birds, no cheerfully chatting people enticed by this sunny Sunday morning to go out for a cycle ride or a walk. You are enclosed in a soundproof box, a statutory requirement to protect your head, which considerably limits your freedom of movement.

You are unaware of the fact that you hear none of these sounds, for this has been completely normal to you since you turned sixteen. The deafening racket from your exhaust pipe boosts your ego, it's all part of the fun. If you can't hear walkers or cyclists approaching, that's not your problem. Let them watch out for themselves! You wear a solid helmet and ride a nice heavy moped.

Taking curves is fun, especially if the road is quiet, which it certainly is on this clear Sunday morning in autumn. Not a soul to be seen or heard. Let it rip! You feel like a real macho, hanging into the curve, what a trip! Man oh man, how sweet it is. The fact that you're hogging the wrong side of the road doesn't interest you. You scrunch up your shoulders, otherwise you'll never get up to speed. Anyway, you're keeping your eyes peeled!

But do you know that taking a sharp curve at much too high speed can cause you to lose control of your moped? In any case, you can no longer solve that problem. You don't manage to steer clear of two cyclists looming up suddenly out of nowhere and heading straight towards you. After all, you can't hear or see a thing.

And, sure enough, you're riding so fast you crash into the nearest cyclist head-on, flinging her into someone's front garden a few yards away, where she lies unconscious.

Now you take off your helmet. It is dead quiet. You could even hear the birds sing, were the silence not disturbed by the harsh noise of rasping, faltering breathing as the unconscious cyclist fights for her life.

The police are soon on the scene and you get booked. An ambulance with shrieking siren takes the unconscious victim to the University Hospital, high-dependency neurology ward. She has brain injury. You ride home on your moped.

I don't send this either.

Recovery

When from one day to the next I found myself saddled with a brain injury, my first thoughts on arriving back home from the hospital were not about treatment in a rehabilitation center. That's something I associated more with visible suffering, with wheelchairs and artificial limbs. Moreover, I had never even heard of brain injury and had no idea what it would mean for me and the people around me. My husband and I were wanderers in the desert, and no one was volunteering to guide us.

But there was one point of light. We knew someone with the recently established National Coordination Center for Non-congenital Brain Damage and via her, in the summer after the accident, I found my way to a rehabilitation center. There, for the first time, I met people who really listened to me.

I was flabbergasted: both the rehabilitation specialist and the psychologist recognized my problems. They were even able to refine the diagnosis. Many of my complaints, they said, suggested a "post-contusional syndrome", as well as a post-whiplash situation.

In retrospect, the reference to whiplash was not so odd. Research shows that contusio cerebri suffered by cyclists is not infrequently found in combination with whiplash injuries. I may well have been a double victim.

The rehabilitation specialist asked to see the x-rays of my back and neck made after the accident. We had to ask the hospital neurology department for them. She also examined my back, neck and shoulders. Strange that no one had done that before. She asked me to bend over and observed that bending my neck even slightly nearly made me fall over and that turning my neck caused me to wobble. Moving still tired me and made me dizzy.

I answered the questions put to me as well as I could. The doctor at the center was actually the first specialist who gave me the time and the peace to express myself. Now and then she nodded. Was that to encourage me or because she had heard these complaints before?

It took me an enormous amount of effort to open the right windows of memory at the right time. My forehead and cheeks were glowing and the situation was becoming unbearable. I broke down and started sobbing.

I could not live in this twilight zone, that's how I saw it. My bruised head was only serviceable for a short time each day. Then I could no longer think and would literally just sit there with an uncontrollable and disobedient body, seeing nothing, and with that fire burning in my face. At such times I could think only of one thing: how can I put out that fire?

When patients are brought unconscious into the hospital after a traffic accident, it is usually impossible for the doctor on duty to come into contact with them. Thus, since he cannot base his diagnosis on complaints from the patient, a standard procedure is followed.

When confronted with an unconscious casualty who is not bleeding anywhere, the doctor examines the knees and hands to determine whether x-rays should be made. Will the victim still be able to move this or that part without pain or not?

I would imagine that the procedure to be followed depends on the type of vehicle the victim was riding or driving. Everyone knows that cyclists have absolutely no protection against a high-speed motorized assault. But are cyclists more extensively examined for this reason?

Ultimately, my non-functionality was completely acknowledged and I heard no more about having to "gradually increase the load". For what is "gradually" and what does "load" mean? For months now I had been running up against, or rather staggering into, my minimal load-bearing capacity.

I evidently feel that the people in the rehabilitation center understand me, because for the first time I am able to take a good hard look at the hand I have been dealt. Without hesitation, I can say that my life since that disastrous accident has been devastated. For the first time since the accident, too, the tears start to flow.

The rehabilitation specialist also seems to sense that despite everything I am still trying to explore my limits. She describes it as a "desperate struggle to prove herself".

Indeed, I seize the slightest excuse to try and stretch myself to the utmost, something I am neither literally nor figuratively able to do. It drives me to despair, and she has grasped that very well. Giving in to limitations is not in my nature. According to the neurologist who first treated me, there was nothing to be seen in the x-rays, so why after eight or nine months could I still only take part to such a limited extent in daily domestic life?

After the rehabilitation specialist, I speak to the rehabilitation psychologist in the center. A man who summons the patience to listen to me and then proposes exhausting tests focusing on visual perception and the ability to distinguish shapes.

Had I not been so closely watched, I might well have thrown in the towel pretty quickly. But this time I make an all-out effort. I am pushed far beyond my capacity.

Once the tests are over, my rehabilitation therapy is proposed, with activities such as swimming, physiotherapy, learning to deal with my changed living conditions and to recognize signals of overexertion. Finally, experiments involving the development of new activities are suggested. Just hearing about them gives me the creeps: handicrafts, watercolors and, even worse, working with clay. I can't bear the thought. Here I am, not yet fifty, and they're trying to keep me occupied like an old lady?

Since then I have learned that there are various forms of rehabilitation. One of these is ambulatory rehabilitation therapy, which I refused for a number of reasons: there were too many people walking around me, it was too crowded and too many activities were offered. Each time I would have to see a different person, would again have to talk and then go back home again.

After my first visit to the rehabilitation center I am reeling on my feet, weary and discouraged. I can't face the idea of yet more tiring and nerve-racking taxi rides, the bother with credit cards and the number I can never remember, the anxious wait to see if the taxi actually comes to pick me up, for where did I put that phone number and what time is he supposed to come anyway?

The doctor is apparently used to all this, for to my relief her reaction is calm and relaxed. In any case, she has always been friendly and understanding. Looking back I realize that you tend to cling to reliable people during a time of recovery and she is definitely one. The only request of mine she cannot fulfil is my wish to remove certain elements from the overall treatment plan. I asked her for speech lessons and lip exercises because my face is terribly stiff and painful. If I want to exercise my tongue I can only do so at the rehabilitation center.

Via Willem I let the rehabilitation specialist know that the proposal to give me outpatient treatment two or three times a week is too demanding for me. "She has a feeling that she does not yet have a clear enough idea of what good it will do her to be an outpatient with you", he explains. "The program that she has already set up for herself at home could be disturbed by your program." And he lists my activities at home: trying to read a bit, looking after the immediate family, as well as keeping things in order in and around the house and cycling. He fears that taking on even more of a load would cause my condition to go from "bad to worse".

The decision to refuse outpatient treatment may sound egocentric, but it is not. My resolve is partly based on the responsibility I feel for my home environment. I am afraid that being absent so frequently will make a complete mess of my attempts at housekeeping. I have just begun to apply my professional experience with so-called programmed instruction to household tasks. Activities I bungle time and time again I have now set out step-by-step in an "idiot's list". In this way, I am developing my own ergotherapy.

After a checkup one year after the accident the rehabilitation specialist writes to the neurologist that I am making very slow progress in terms of concentration and memory. That I avoid crowds and commotion and like to be outside as much as possible. Only with my husband do I still undertake a few light activities and then only on familiar ground.

Nonetheless, I still frequently suffer from splitting headaches. Certain movements drive me stark raving mad. And I am very easily irritated. In conclusion, my situation is described as "extremely unstable".

The rehabilitation specialist is gravely concerned about my mental resilience. She notes: "There is still the possibility of serious depression".

Phew!

Eighteen months after the accident, following the checkup by the rehabilitation specialist, I have a long talk with the psychologist. He clearly points out the traps I should avoid and I try to think of concrete examples drawn from my daily life. It is impossible to avoid thinking that I will never manage it, or that if I do my marriage and family life will go completely on the rocks!

Thanks to my old profession, public administration and management consultancy, I am familiar with the concepts of structure and strategy. But the idea that they may also be of benefit to the rehabilitation process is new to me. I must integrate an effective structure and useful strategies into my daily life.

Learn to set yourself limits is the message. But with a heavy heart I know that to me this is a huge amputation of my personality and temperament. And how am I supposed to come to terms with it?

My progress that year was described by the rehabilitation center as "very slight". My adaptability was said to be "reasonably good". Yet the rehabilitation specialist again thinks that a "reactive depression" may be lying in wait for me.

Speech therapy has been proposed to improve my control over the movements of my mouth and reduce the pain in my face and head. But this can only be arranged for me within the walls of the rehabilitation center. And since I don't want that, nothing is done about it.

Looking back, I can think of various examples characterizing the successive phases of my recovery. If I dig deep in my memory, which is still an exhausting task, I can find a few significant situations appearing in little clouds of recollection: my stay in the University Hospital, the first six weeks at home, walks in the park, visits to the Other Party's insurers, visits to the Medical Examination Service and the rehabilitation center.

These examples probably remained in my memory because they involved "failure behavior". In healthy situations, a normal dose of such failure behavior can be compensated for by positive experiences. You don't need to display "avoidance behavior" because you have enough energy to enable the number of positive experiences to prevail over the negative. Following contusio cerebri, however, there is no longer any question of this. There is a chronic lack of energy to confront all the challenges raised by the problems related to orientation in time and space.

So what I do is very selectively expose myself to these problems. And each time I am again surprised that a problem still exists. Thus it becomes more and more difficult to make progress, no matter how slight, and the urge to avoid such energy-draining problems with their far-reaching dreadfully tiring consequences becomes greater and greater. Other things come first. The housekeeping must continue, and I must and will keep managing the kitchen. That takes all my energy.

An initial memory (orientation in time).

After a visit to the rehabilitation center, I ask the receptionist to call a taxi to take me home. It takes too much effort for me to exchange information on my feet. I am dizzy, I look like the Leaning Tower of Pisa. Last time the psychologist called a taxi for me, this time I have to do it myself.

I sit in the reception area and wait, looking around me as little as possible to curtail the stimuli produced by passing wheelchairs. A sluggish toneless voice makes an announcement. A pretty young girl, apparently undamaged, sits down in the waiting room too. I look the other way. The taxi is still keeping me waiting.

How long it takes I have no idea. I no doubt look at my watch, but can't keep the time in mind. But I sit there patiently. Until one of the receptionists comes up to me and asks: "Haven't you been picked up yet?"

They have forgotten me. Now she goes back to the telephone, keeping an eye on me until I am finally picked up.

Another memory (orientation in space).

"Do you know the way to my house?" With Femke, my right-hand woman, I am walking through our neighborhood park. She keeps a firm hold on my arm. We need a half-hour to cover a stretch that used to take me ten minutes. I keep having to stand still because everything goes gray before my eyes. It is almost impossible to utter a word because moving forward demands all my concentration.

I expressly call it moving forward and not walking. Moving forward involves much, much more: watching out for holes in the path that might cause me to fall, avoiding dog dirt, making sure I don't run into low-hanging branches. I have already more or less broken the habit of deciding whether or not to greet the people who pass me on the path.

I much prefer it if nobody talks to me. Most people walk in the park to be seen and spoken too, with or without their dogs, but not me. I am here to practice the technique of forward motion in its most complex form.

There is much more to it than I had thought. My concentration is focused on walking, keeping my balance, and not constantly stumbling! But on the way back I suddenly can't see the wood for the trees. I've forgotten the way to my own house.

Can't we just ask someone? I won't hear of it, my independence knows no bounds. We'll manage somehow. "Femke", I say, "just be quiet, let me think!" I know that we have to get to an open space, after that it's simple. And in the end we succeed.

Once back home I collapse on the couch, dead tired and speechless. Are we still having fun? No. Femke makes lunch, but I just wish she would go home. I'm no use to anyone now. All I want is peace and quiet.

In his book, *The Cerebral Symphony*, William H. Calvin writes: "The pre-motor cortex specializes in setting up sequences of actions, as when you insert a key into the lock, turn the doorknob, and finally push open the door. Patients with damage only to left premotor cortex will be able to perform each action separately—there is no inability to move, as in motor strip injuries —but will have difficulty chaining the actions together into a fluent motion, what Luria called a 'kinetic melody'."

Calvin states that "premotor" problems can lead to difficulties in switching from one rhythm to the other.

I know what he's talking about from my own experience.

One more example from my gradual recovery process. When I come home and open the front door with the key, my legs stop working. I have to put down my bag and walk through the hall to the alarm on legs moving slow as molasses, even though it seems to me that I'm rushing as fast as I can. During the first few months after the accident I always arrived at the alarm too late, so that the big siren began to shriek. My husband couldn't understand it at all. "Just walk a bit faster!" With a series of actions incomprehensible to me he shuts down the siren.

Later comes the phase where I do manage to get to the keyboard in time but have absolutely no idea which keys I am meant to press. The note with the code gives me little comfort. It is still difficult to translate the note into action on the keyboard. It takes me too long to figure it out.

Finally the last phase dawns. I even know the new code by heart! That's because I made it up myself, with the help of a memory aid.

Five years after the accident I still have problems with the transition from cycling to walking. I trip over everything in my way, in the first place of course my bicycle. Despite my long legs, I have set the saddle as low as possible. Being able to put both feet on the ground when braking makes it easier to get off and prevents wobbling. First I hold the bicycle calmly between both legs, then get off, with the cycle to one side.

But then my legs refuse to walk. I have to wait for them for quite some time before they listen to me again and I stumble jerkily forwards. Their protest continues awhile before finally vanishing imperceptibly.

Needless to say all this only turns out well when I am alone. As soon as I am distracted, there is a greater risk of falling and a disproportionate increase in fatigue.

A person can get used to anything, even waiting for her legs. But I still get angry and annoyed when Willem yells at me: "What's keeping you?"

I know that he can't see anything wrong with me, but I still think there's no excuse for his impatience. I expect him to be observant, and preferably silent!

But from whom can I demand such an attitude? Even professionals have disappointed me in this regard. And blowing my stack about it would be a senseless waste of energy.

I still have so much to learn.

The experts at the rehabilitation center persuade me that I should stand up for myself better, assert myself to protect my interests. Be egocentric is their motto. I don't like that word, but I am up to my eyes in misery and it is obvious that something has to change. I can't keep stumbling along like a zombie forever. What can I do differently?

In the daytime I keep my front door locked to prevent surprise visits. I find it repugnant and unnatural to lock myself up like a prisoner in my own home, but it turns out to be a healthy decision. At first, people seem surprised. "You shouldn't shut yourself up like that, it's not good for you." But in fact it is very good for me. My home has become an impenetrable fortress so that I again have my hands free to relearn the basic housekeeping skills.

Although still plagued by great fatigue and many pains, I again have a flicker of hope. Little by little, I am expanding my training ground beyond the front door. And with many (literal) ups and downs, I am enlarging my habitat in slow motion. With one condition that is very new to me: I do everything on my own. Even though time after time I receive friendly offers to undertake various activities with old friends or neighbors, I learn to say no, initially with pain in my heart.

Once in a while I "sin", but then I am so heavily flattened by a general malaise and severe headaches lasting two to three days that I realize the price was too high.

I go through bottomless pits I can't share with anyone, for then I am invariably advised to "come on over" or "give us a call". But human beings have a wide range of chameleonic qualities enabling them to more or less deal with a changed life.

I now have three concrete objectives:
- Posture: by means of specific exercises, interspersed with rest periods, I intend to go from nearly 100% horizontal to at least 90% vertical in the daytime.
- Through a process of habituation and adaptation, I want to be able to participate as fully as possible in social life again.
- Using material appropriate to my level and interests, I want to expand my reading, writing and speaking skills.

To achieve these objectives, my homemade treatment plan focuses on three elements:
- My capacity for forward movement in all imaginable household situations and subsequently outside as well.

- My bruised head, which has great difficulty making observations, distinctions, plans and decisions, and also suffers from impaired orientation in time and space.
- My social life, inextricably linked with the social life of my husband and sons.

This is my approach to recovery.

Life With The Brakes On

In principle, people are social animals. There is even a special word for people who withdraw from society and not only live on their own but also renounce the comforts of modern life: hermits.

People look on them as oddballs, pity them a little, maybe even find them a bit pathetic. After all, communication with others is a fully accepted, normally satisfied need. If a child rejects all forms of communication, he or she will soon be under investigation. That is... abnormal.

As I write this, I am having a slight problem finding the right word, a slight touch of ...aphasia. The little window in my brain won't open up. What do they call this non-communicative behavior again? Dyslexia? Aphasia? No, those words are both wrong. But they sound very much like the word I'm looking for.

Formerly friends tell me Latin terms simply tripped off my tongue, and in the right context. Now it takes more than half an hour before I connect the non-communicative child with the term "autism" in my brain.

Is it possible to examine how that "search function" works? Did I make use of specific efficient strategies to pry that jammed rusty shutter open?

What I did in this case was to search via Latin sounds, while simultaneously images flashed through my head of a kid who looked past me, made no eye contact and sat crouched in a corner. Then, in the wink of an eye, the word appeared. I wrote down the sentence: "It took more than half an hour before..." and the word had vanished again!

My brain plays tricks on me. I forgot that when I find a word I must immediately, but really immediately, write it down. I no longer remembered that I don't function as I used to anymore.

It takes me an incredible amount of energy to get this kind of cognitive thought process going. It takes brainwork, and heavy concentration. It is literally like racking my brains.

In a conversation I would not have bothered, for I cannot simultaneously search for a word and follow a discussion. But even when I am writing by myself in total peace and calm, the act of thinking creates such great pressure on my head and forehead that it is still very unpleasant.

If there were some technique for registering where this search strategy starts my cerebral links glowing red-hot, would this provide more insight into the size of the scorched spots in relation to the scale of the brain injury? My brain feels like a glowing coal, a stiff, sticky, burning feeling. A color photo would speak volumes.

I have to go do something else for awhile, pick up branches in the garden or something like that, to avoid being bowled over by that strange, oppressive head. It's raining cats and dogs but out I go anyway, in sou'wester and rain boots. It does my head good.

What is actually so essential about the need for community and communication? In the western world, young people are conditioned by their upbringing and education into socially desirable products: people who communicate, negotiate and make choices. The language with which to communicate and the free will to decide are our most valuable attributes, distinguishing human beings from animals.

As a result of the brain injury, my possibilities for making use of this most human and accepted means of expression, language, have been seriously impaired. My educational ideal ("Put all your energy into self-development, for possessions can always be lost") has turned out to be extremely vulnerable and now seems built on sand.

What a silly goose I was. Who could have suspected that there are scoundrels on the roads who can devastate this most essential and personal realm without so much as a by-your-leave or a slap on the wrist?

Or was I blissfully unaware? Of course I knew that people are struck down by tumors, strokes and all kinds of degenerative diseases. But it had never occurred to me that you could suffer brain injury through the fault of another.

Before the accident my aim was to "acquire knowledge through unending education". Acquiring brain injury was not part of the program.

Now I have acquired brain injury, but it is thanks to another person that I have acquired it.

People have different talents. One has golden hands, renovates his own house down to the tiniest detail, the other has a creative bent and knits cardigan after cardigan in the most complicated patterns. People always said about me that I had the gift of gab. Many doors opened up for me. In tricky situations I always managed to think of something to say to save the day. You could safely leave it to me to develop contacts at many different levels.

The fact that I had this capacity I only fully realized after the accident, when I became totally incapable of doing it anymore. Before it had been so obvious that I didn't even mention it. Colleagues used to say I had a broad perspective on a number of areas and I supported this with lots of reading and writing. My wide-ranging interests needed a good deal of sustenance. Moreover, I must have had boundless energy, for the concept of "early to bed" was alien to me. I hated to go to sleep, found it a waste of time.

Now the people around me comfort me by pointing out that we all forget a word from time to time, for "we're all getting older day by day". It took me a long time to stop getting angry at so much lack of understanding. Can't they see that my forgetting is of an entirely different kind, if only because of the cause and the frequency with which it occurs?

I have resolved to stop trying to explain the difference. It takes too much energy and makes no impression anyway.

The longer a conversation lasts, the more problems I have finding the right words. I falter and stammer more too. The sentences stick in my throat. I become more and more dizzy and groggy. My brain flashes "tilt" like a pinball machine run amuck. The only solution is to be by myself in silence.

The fact that I am forced to terminate communication costs me dearly in terms of persuasiveness and expressiveness. Not only am I unsteady on my feet, but the balance of power in my life has also been knocked askew.

Could writing soften the blow somewhat?

In any case, it's worth trying. Making the most of my time is becoming more and more of a problem. I will have to use the satisfaction I get from it as a new source of energy to keep to this path I have taken.

A void that cannot be filled has been created by the departure of neighbors who have divorced and moved away. Our children went to nursery and primary school together, played sports together, before fanning out in different directions. That produced a bond that has now been suddenly cut. And there is nothing to replace it.

A man with a brain injury would probably have less difficulty with this kind of thing. In general, it is the wife who is responsible for the social side of life, along with looking after the household management. For me, the absence of these old familiar faces comes as a hard blow. We weren't always knocking on each other's door, but we were there for each other when necessary. When I cycle past their house now, there is no one to say hello to anymore.

There is a growing sense of anonymity. I'm in a miserable situation.

The accident has had a nasty effect on my temper. If anyone gets in my way I fly into a rage. I make bitter remarks, curse everything and everyone, vent my fury verbally at the people around me. "Leave me alone, you're driving me nuts! Don't talk to me! Beat it!"

Anyone who still tries to tell me something gets the full blast. So children and husband, keep your heads down. All I want is Peace Peace Peace. Don't make any kind of racket or I'll really hit the ceiling.

I mean it. I have been transformed into an unreasonable hit-the-ceiling kind of person. If someone points out to me, reproachfully or not, that dinner isn't ready yet or there are no more clean shirts in the closet I burst into tears. Can't they see something's wrong with me? Don't these louts notice that I'm not functioning properly?

Even those closest to me look surprised when I say I can't do something or go somewhere on my own. I have changed into a silly old biddy who gets angry at remarks like "Can't you manage that? Are you afraid of falling?"

I boil with rage at so much lack of understanding. And if I try to say a few venomous words back, at my old rapid pace, then something happens I never experienced before: I start stuttering.

I feel very much alone, isolated and misunderstood.

After such confrontations I need about five hours alone to cool down my head. After that I can again cautiously walk around the house before settling down to sleep.

In Training

It often takes years for traffic casualties to free themselves from fear. Time after time I am confronted with 'strange' feelings in traffic. My heart pounds, I can't catch my breath, I become very emotional, angry, or rather furious, sometimes I weep from impotence. When do I get so upset? When do I start shaking like a leaf? Every time this happens to me, cycling on my own or with Willem, my anxiety attacks are triggered by mopeds. Incomprehensible! That I should be so affected when I remember nothing at all of the actual accident! Speeding moped riders three abreast, hogging the whole road. A moped racing on the cycle path in the woods (no mopeds allowed), suddenly swerving towards a couple of hikers. They all had one thing in common: they were coming towards me.

I don't panic easily, so there's no question of that, but I do transform into a whining puppy.

The terror of oncoming traffic has me in its grip not only on my bicycle but also in the car. Each time a vehicle comes towards me riding on or over the center line on the highway it scares me stiff, stupefies me. The thought of an accident obsesses me. Each time I feel a deadly crash heading my way caused by the reckless behavior of the oncoming driver and have no idea how to arm myself against these budding traffic criminals.

This fear came over me for the first time when Willem picked me up at the hospital. "Don't drive so darned fast!" I yelled at him on the highway. He looked at me with surprise: "I'm not driving fast at all!" I was doubtful, because I had the feeling that the cars were whizzing past. Months later I read that Loe De Jong had the same experience after his cerebral hemorrhage. He too complained when his wife picked him up at the hospital: "How ridiculously fast all these cars are going!"

I tell the community health service doctor about my strategy for overcoming my self-diagnosed phobia. Not avoidance but confrontation. Little by little. Not so hard in overpopulated Holland, where you are confronted with mopeds at every street corner whether you like it or not. He listens and is amazed at my personal approach, which he supports.

But what good does that do me? I want help. What more can I do? After all, he's the one who sees hordes of contusio cerebri traffic casualties pass by his desk. How do they recover, on the whole? Can he give me some kind of prognosis?

For why am I telling him this whole story? Because, practically without seeing me, he wants me to pursue a course of behavioral therapy. He notes down the name of a psychologist for me in case I have more problems. The word 'depression' is not spoken, but I feel it hanging in the air.

I get more out of physiotherapy. The first physiotherapist made his appearance in our lives when Willem was flattened by acute back pain shortly before Christmas the year following my accident. He couldn't walk at all anymore, could only lie down with the help of injections of painkillers. Willem called the district nursing service, which provided him with a chamber pot and a bottle, essential accessories for bed-bound patients.

The elderly man who came to deliver these items saw a relatively young and healthy woman open the door for him. I found it necessary to explain that I had a brain injury and was thus unable to drive to a place I had never been before to pick them up myself. Moreover, now that my husband was out of action I was stressed to the limit. Our home office, which normally had its own entrance, had now been moved to the living and dining room. All day long, phone and fax lines were ringing and Willem was beeping and clicking away on his laptop. The peace in my home had utterly vanished, what with all the care-givers coming and going, not to mention my husband's friends, all of whom he had by now informed.

It was precisely the worst possible environment for me. I was closer to tears than to laughter. Meanwhile Willem's doctor visited him almost daily. And when Willem at last with much moaning and groaning got to his feet again, his upper body appeared to be considerably out of line with his lower. It was hard not to laugh. Two cripples under one roof!

But Willem couldn't see the humor in it. His doctor referred him to a physiotherapy center to get him moving again. A young therapist came to our house to 'manipulate' him and soon had Willem back on his feet to the point where he could drive to the physiotherapy center himself.

What a lovely profession, I thought, and what a miracle that results are achieved so quickly.

The physiotherapist turned out to be a sharp observer. With amazement, he closely watched my slow waddling movements around the house. No doubt I had closed my own eyes to it. When he heard what I had, he offered his services with conviction. He believed his treatment would make things somewhat better for me.

How amusing, I thought, such a young man and so sure of himself. I would ask the neurologist, I said, for secretly I was afraid that a small crack or slight fracture in my back and neck vertebrae might have been missed in the x-rays. So I wanted his approval.

Then I read a book about various forms of treatment to find out where physiotherapy stood in relation to conventional medicine and how physiotherapists were trained. I read that practitioners of physiotherapy and physical medicine accepted the same 'concepts of disease' current in conventional medicine. That clinched it for me. Weird alternative therapies had cost a brother of mine his life.

Willem admonished the therapist once more to handle me very carefully, considering the whiplash injury I might have. And then we could begin.

Nearly a year and a half after the accident I drove the car to the physiotherapist for the first time, my sole activity of the day. My case history was noted down with painstaking precision. It was very soon evident that the physical examination I would be subjected to would be a combination of orthopedic functional investigation, neurological examination and physical medical examination. No question of strange herbal brews or vague and wooly explanations. On the contrary, I was in the hands of someone with a thorough knowledge of everything that had to do with the locomotor apparatus. The spinal column, the head, the neck, the chest, the lumbar region, the pelvis and the limbs, he was privy to all their secrets.

I had come to the right place. My aches and pains, jerky locomotor functions and problems with balance were finally getting the attention and care they had so long gone without. Without the slightest hesitation he designated my super-stiff and painful areas by their Latin names. That inspired great confidence in me. He also took seriously my restricted movements, which were often accompanied by unpleasant tingling sensations.

What followed was a lengthy but very worthwhile treatment. We began with two sessions a week, but it soon became evident that once a week was enough for me. And thanks to the exercises I had to do at home, the treatment wasn't restricted to passively receiving 'manipulations' for an hour a week.

When I lay stretched out on the treatment table it was utterly impossible for me to lift up my head. Well, ten pounds is quite heavy after all. My neck seemed to be a big hard hunk of steel, totally impervious to the command 'lift head'. So next to nothing happened. Sitting on the table, it appeared that the slightest movement of my head caused my arms to fly up as aids to keep me from falling off the table.

Later I was given active exercise therapy aimed at increasing the mobility of my neck. The 'homework' I was given initially gave me great difficulty, for I only remembered two of the five exercises.

At a later stage I had to train my sense of balance by sitting on a large ball. I also had to bounce and catch a ball while walking. Despite being able to sit and relax during the break, at the end of the session I staggered out of the center like a drunk.

Nearly three years after the accident I carefully started playing tennis again, fifteen-minute sessions against the wall at the neighbors across the street. Consequences: headache, dizziness and walking drunkenly.

A year later I went twice a week for a half-hour each time. My forehead began to feel better. At the start of the season my head ached terribly and I was exhausted at the end of a session. These symptoms disappeared after a few weeks. On condition that I took enough rest and did not let the post-tennis euphoria tempt me to answer the telephone or even call someone up myself to talk about how well things were going with me and the progress I was making. This temptation was great, but if I yielded to it I suffered the consequences almost as soon as I put down the phone. I was punished for such 'splurges' with severe headaches and a staggering gait. This was my greatest handicap, for I have a tremendous urge to communicate.

Meanwhile knocking tennis balls against the neighbors' wall gave me a great deal of satisfaction and I was content with what was still possible for me. And besides it made me more cheerful. This activity had a fourfold goal: increasing blood circulation to the brain, training in hand-eye coordination, exercising my legs and improving my balance by moving sideways and backwards.

The physiotherapist starts me on tennis ball therapy three and a half years after my accident. Bouncing the ball on the ground, against the wall and on the tennis racket. They are dreadful exercises that make me dizzy and sick as a dog.

Sometimes I am very close to tears, but I don't cry. I get fed up with myself, think I am demanding the impossible, that things will never change, and refuse to practice anymore. I have reached my limit. I hate this therapy and never want to come back, even though I don't say so. I look ridiculous , keep falling over, can't take a normal step anymore and still have to make my way home. I feel like a lonely and misunderstood fool.

But the following week I drive calmly back to the center, for am I a weakling who gives up at the slightest setback? No. I buckle down to work again, motivated by the thought that progress is better than standing still. I must do what I can, so that later I won't have to say "if only I had tried harder".

Lydie comes to see if I can run fast enough to play in the old tennis club again. Sometimes I join in for an hour, usually when I don't have to look after my husband or children that evening, so that I can be sure of being left in peace afterwards. I also sit down during the break when gossip is shared. The dizzy feeling vanishes when I sit on a chair on the terrace. It doesn't trouble me in the car on the way home either. I do get dizzy on the bicycle, especially when crossing intersections and looking over my shoulder. For the time being, therefore, I have to use the car to travel even that short way.

My handicaps when playing tennis are that I get dizzy when serving and often lose track of where I am supposed to hit the ball. Actually, I should wait to serve until I am standing solidly on my two feet, for aiming the ball precisely demands a great deal of cerebral coordination and puts a strain on my neck.

Picking up tennis balls, especially when they're rolling, exhausts me and makes me dizzy. I use the tried and tested foot-racket method to avoid bending over as much as possible. My old tennis partner Willemien is clearly aware that I have trouble with this and regularly picks up my balls for me and shows me the spot where I am supposed to serve (underhand). She also acts as my umpire, for she is better than anyone at keeping my score, something I regularly get wrong.

After a lot of practice, I begin to recover my old feeling for the ball as well as my strong forehand, a gratifying result both for me and my opponents.

And so I struggle slowly up to speed again. My attempts to play on the indoor courts as well still lead inevitably to a splitting headache. The clamor from the nearby courts combined with the fast-moving players swarming all around have a troublesome effect on me that is hard to shake off.

When cycling I always take the same routes, making it virtually impossible to get lost. I started in the traffic-free woods, and now I can cycle to the center of our busy little town. A milestone.

In September, nearly four years after the accident, I started fitness training in a sports center near my home under the guidance of a man-and-wife team of physiotherapists. First I had to take a test, based on my pulse rate, after which the physiotherapist, having determined my height, weight and age, arrived at the following diagnosis: you are at the start of the fitness ladder. The first rung. That made sense, since I had had to stop taking the first-rung test before it was over. In bold type, the computer printout proclaimed that I had a 'greatly diminished capacity'. The conclusion: you have an acute lack of fitness. And what's more: the extent to which you are unfit greatly increases your risk of serious cardiovascular disease.

I am assigned to the lowest level and to score my weekly points I am allowed to rotate between three machines. But the last thing I want is to switch machines. It is deadly tiring and gives me problems with dizziness and decision-making. Furthermore, it is impossible for me to fathom three systems in a single go, with all those computers and scores you have to somehow keep an eye on.

To begin with, my tactic is to keep track of one or at most two bits of data on the screen: the points to be scored and the average speed I must try to maintain. I literally shut my eyes to the rest. Looking for these two things on the screen is quite tiring enough.

The exercise bike tells me I am now cycling around five and a half miles in a half an hour, an average of 11 miles an hour, often with my eyes closed and hands free. This is only possible here. I can't reach such speeds on the road, for one thing because it would give me problems with 'reading' the environment. If I want to keep up this pace, I am condemned to the indoor fitness center for the time being.

Each week, I must score a minimum of 8 and a maximum of 11 points on the cardiovascular machines. I am advised that it would be best to come three times a week. The trainer wants me to improve my condition not only on the exercise bike but also on the treadmill and rowing machine. He is positive about my athletic medical curve, which indicates a gradual increase in heartbeat from 85 to 145. I have fitness level 1, a euphemism for someone who fails to finish the test due to exhaustion.

The results of a half-hour on the exercise bike are twofold. In the first place, I summon the energy to drive over there around three-thirty in the afternoon and give myself some relaxation and distraction at a time when I am otherwise not up to much. The second and most important result, however, is a lightening of the pressure on my head, particularly my forehead, which always becomes more and more rigid in the course of the day, especially after talking. This relief is not definitive, but it does last a few hours, on condition that I refrain from talking.

Could there be some benefit from intensifying blood circulation in the head and spine? Some neurologists believe this is a fairytale. But when such relief can be generated from intensive training on the exercise bike, you certainly get addicted. Then three times a week is definitely no punishment.

The first week I did it I had severe lower back pain, but perseverance again won out. Even when I hadn't exercised for two weeks, I no longer suffered pain, so I simply kept going, on to the next level.

The treadmill and the rowing machine, which I also could have used, I left alone for the time being.

Will I really be able to move up a rung on the fitness ladder? Previously (I shouldn't compare but I like to anyway), I used to do fitness dance till I practically dropped, but I never had headaches. On what fitness rung will I now have to stand to be able to function at that level? In terms of coordination and stamina it seems a totally unreachable goal to me.

After nearly six months I am halfway to rung 2. The system has me in its grasp. There is no need to talk to anyone. I can restrict my conversations to the bare essentials. I now spend an hour on the machines up to three times a week. In any case it keeps me busy, even during the afternoons, when my spine has the tendency to cave in and my forehead feels like a rigid board.

After a workout I have a delightfully clean feeling in my lungs and forehead that I am becoming addicted to.

It took me a long time before I was able to adjust the computers on the machines to my personal data. I had great difficulty with all the numbers scrolling down the screens. And when it came to entering numbers I hardly knew where to start. For months I restricted myself to a single machine.

Luckily the physiotherapist at the center was kind enough to help me through my rather long 'apraxia'. I use this word because it covers all my problems: remembering and entering different numbers for each machine, distinguishing between the maximum and minimum burden on my heart. Then there were the different keyboards: where do I enter my maximum and minimum numbers on each one? Checking the monitor. And when you have finally found what you want, pressing the right buttons to call up the next command.

By the end of the year I have overcome this apraxia as well. Even though it costs me a good deal of effort to manage the necessary hand-eye coordination. Often I am forced to limit myself to one or two machines, depending on the state of my head.

We are in Andalusia, golfing at Los Naranjos, a lovely club with an equally lovely clubhouse. Due to the rainy weather and the wet ground, it is forbidden to use an electric golf cart. I make a deal with Willem: you pull my handcart or I go home (even though I don't know how I'm going to get there). So Willem pulls my cart.

Afterwards I have no back or neck pain, just fidgety, tingling legs and head. Although it is officially taboo, during the game I keep asking Willem which club I should use. Judging the distance has become extra hard, if not impossible, for me.

Groggy and dizzy, I try not to lose my balance. Sometimes I almost vanish behind the ball. We play a foursome with a Swedish couple. When the wife begins to chat sociably about their trip in the rain to a mountain village and says that she doesn't play much due to her work, I tell her right away that I can't talk and walk at the same time because of a brain injury caused by a traffic accident.

I am glad that the truth is out, otherwise I would have had to keep looking for a suitable moment. That would have taken all the energy I needed simply to keep my balance.

It is still quite pleasant. They chatter away with Willem, who is already beginning to get used to his role as mediator. When Willem forgets she pulls my cart, then looks after the flag and picks up my ball without making me feel inordinately cared for.

I get more and more tired and want to sit down. It had to be today that electric carts are banned. Just my luck. In the old days I wouldn't have fretted about it. Walking is good for the health. Now I'd give anything to ride in a little electric cart. When you have trouble walking and keeping your balance you wind up automatically in the category of old fogies with infirmities. Nowadays I can only do eighteen holes sitting in the cart. And even then I keep bumping my head or hips getting in and out of the thing, especially during the last nine holes.

What an old duffer I have become.

Someone on another fairway hits a ball that lands right next to me with a thump. With no shout of 'fore'—the guy doesn't seem to know the rules— his ball whizzes past, nearly grazing my head. So I stamp that ball with my foot as hard as I can into the ground. Just let it lie, and do the old disappearing act.

My handicap is that I can't keep track of how many strokes I've had, let alone those of my partners. I don't write anything down and always have trouble keeping up the pace. On a new course I can't remember where the holes are. I am forced to rely on others to find the next hole.

A Life Alone?

I must learn to hold my own, even under difficult circumstances. So I have to practice.

That one of my practice situations happens to be a silver wedding anniversary tells you something about our age and that of our best friends, Femke and Lodewijk. Femke manages to talk me into passing up the coffee klatch at their home, but not the lunch. As soon as I arrive at the reception hall I plop myself down on a chair. Around me at least fifty people are waiting to go into the dining room. Some of them come up to me and give me a warm hug. One or two ask how I am. I answer, 'Fine, thanks!'

This part I had rehearsed with Femke beforehand.

Then Femke comes to get me, gives me a big hug and leads me through the crowd to a quiet spot. Two of Femke's sisters sit down next to me. Luckily they know about my accident and its consequences. Femke had also warned me to bring earplugs against the noise.

I am always surprised when people are happy to see me, for what have I got to offer anyone? Don't ask me. When I am in the midst of a large group of people, I squeeze my eyes to tiny slits, focus them on the ground and start lurching along in the desired direction. I know where I want to go, but actually getting there is not so easy.

If I get drawn into conversation as I'm moving around, my clumsy body is bound to stumble straight into a lamp or open door. This old Auntie Slowcoach needs space and silence around her.

Since space and silence are in short supply at this party, I am taken in hand by a friendly sister-in-law.

Despite my gratefulness for this gesture, I still begin to get irritated, even though I don't immediately show it.

Poor Maurits has to take it on the chin when he stops me and asks 'Still remember me?' Even I am shocked by my reply. 'Of course I do—I'm not crazy you know!' I try to make it up to him by kissing him on both cheeks.

I enjoy the party at a distance. During the speeches I now and then take the plugs out of my ears. I tell Roosmarie she has bad luck sitting next to me at the table, for it is impossible for me to say anything through the hubbub around us. I can't hear anything and can't find the words to express myself. The words all seem to be stuck somewhere out of reach, the right words and expressions simply don't come to me.

It takes the utmost concentration for me to be able to listen, let alone speak. The effort is out of all proportion with the simplicity of the conversation, but I won't let myself be frustrated by my own personality that would like nothing better than a rapid exchange of information with all and sundry. I limit myself to a single topic, in this case the excellent cuisine of the restaurant we're in, and make the best of it.

I also enjoy the speeches, and the presence of Femke and Lodewijk's elderly parents. And last but not least the loving remarks of their children. With a joke here and a witty comment there they keep us all laughing.

I begin to get the hang of repressing my old temperament. When someone asks me 'Have you ever been to the States?' I answer 'Yes'. Period. End of topic. Over and out.

'How is your youngest son doing?' 'Fine.' Period. End of topic. Over and out.

As soon as I start to talk at length about anything, my forehead and cheeks suffer inexplicable neurological spasms of pain. If I decide to hang tough and ignore them, the top of my head starts burning too, followed by increasing pressure on head and ears. Until all I can do is lie down somewhere quiet, and that is not always possible. At this silver wedding anniversary, for example, it's absolutely out of the question.

Naturally I try to find out why conversations always result in a hefty dose of pain. Under which circumstances is the situation bearable and when does the pain phase start up, when does that zombie business begin, when do I turn into a ball of fire? Even practicing neurologists have no answers to these questions. Evidently I will have to look after myself.

Creating more favorable circumstances is the way I find most attractive. But how do I go about doing that?

Many people think they can comfort you by saying things like 'I can't do three things at once either'. Unfortunately, they take a much too optimistic view of my situation.

I discover that my problems are taken seriously in the book *Veranderd leven* ('Changed Life') by remedial educationalist Jenny Palm. She states that people with traumatic brain injury have to deal not only with memory disorders but also with attention deficits. According to her, problems with focusing attention arise in the following situations. In the first place, whenever you have to do more than one thing at a time. Talking to someone while you're cooking, or watching a movie and reading subtitles.

Consolation is often offered in words such as these: 'Going to receptions and birthday parties, who gives a hoot about that? They're not so much fun anyway!' But what people forget is that they are part of normal social life. Fortunately, Palm has recognized this problem. The second situation she names is 'crowded conditions'. She gives three examples: birthday parties, receptions, groups. Even today, I still know very well what she is talking about.

Up to now, the only thing that makes any difference for me is when such events are held outside. Then, if I have a chair and don't need to exchange much information, I can hold out for quite some time. But even then, the last thing I need is for some friendly soul to sit down next to me and start an animated conversation. With a chair it's not easy to move somewhere else. You're a captive audience.

With me, however, problems also crop up in my own home:

- After some time I have to flee my husband and children for a peaceful room in the house or a restful spin on my bicycle.
- After explaining the work to be done to my housekeeper, whether verbally or in writing, I need to be alone in a separate, quiet room.
- From the fact that the doorbell keeps ringing I deduce that the note on the door stating where callers should ring is not being read. People are always showing up to carry out repairs on the house, wash the windows, check the central heating, gas, lighting or electricity, and if you don't arrange things perfectly you will be constantly disturbed.

I still cannot bear excessive information exchange. I have to limit my communication periods, dose them out as precisely as the ingredients for an exquisite recipe. That's something you decide in advance, it is the secret agenda.

Anyone who surprises me during my quiet times and faces my resentment at a sudden visit, no matter how short, is unintentionally making light of my handicap. I cannot react flexibly to unexpected visits because it already takes so much verbal effort just to say politely: 'Not right now, please'.

Even with close friends, what works best for me is to chat a little every day. If I haven't spoken to him for a week I have problems even with Willem and have to flee to my bed very early. I stammer and can't get the words out, become dizzy and drowsy.

Variation exhausts me and takes far too much energy.

I look through the lonely hearts ads to practice reading. What tiresome reading matter. But the recalcitrant brain needs practice and there are plenty of ads to read. Travel, concerts, nightlife, that's what everyone wants. Nowhere do I see: 'Good-natured hermit writer seeks like-minded partner who also wants to live together but still on her own. Gardening, reading and cooking are absolute musts.'

It seems impossible to keep avoiding communication. The pressure from the family is already considerable and if you add on outside obligations I would be bouncing like an aimless ball from one interaction to the next with neighbors and friends.

But isn't that nice and sociable? No. Not if you feel like I do after a little chat on the sidewalk.

The more often it happens, the less I can do in a day, and the more I feel like a windup toy handed over to my dizzy brain. Each communication is a flow of information back and forth. The greater the flow, the worse my head reacts to it. Until finally I can't do anything anymore, can't bear anyone near me, am dead tired and sluggish and laborious in everything I do, plagued by the pressure in my head and my unmanageable arms and legs.

If only I was not such a social animal, I would now lead an easier life.

August in the Alps is a festive time. I walk to a house where a concert is to be given. The last stretch is quite steep and my untrained calves protest. Naturally I have taken the longer and wider path up the mountain. There is little rocky ground to stumble over, so it is the ideal route for me.

Since it is late in the afternoon, I have taken my walking stick with me, my third leg that gives me more stability. I stand still now and then to delight in the environment, a marvelous panorama of snowy four-thousand-meter peaks.

Gasping I reach the sitting room where the concert will take place. Willem, swift as a young hound, is already there. He is sitting in the front row winking enthusiastically at me, happy that I am again going to a concert with him.

I make it through the first half-hour reasonably well. The tones of the violin penetrate deeply into me. I listen intensely and can distinguish the different tempos.

Then suddenly my forehead begins to tingle and my cheeks join in too. The music becomes a devilish din in my ears. The moment has come to put in my earplugs. Luckily I have them with me. Bringing earplugs to a home concert? Everyone can see me putting them in, but I could care less. The muffled tones give blessed relief to the tingling in my head.

Of course I am also sitting too close to the music, but I couldn't find a seat further back. From now on I must keep my distance more and above all not be so groundlessly optimistic.

What I am doing now is listening to music as a social occasion. The time of intense listening and enjoyment is over, I have to take a step backwards.

Nonetheless, I am happy with my relative progress, since for the first time I don't feel like howling with pain. I am in the tolerance phase: the music glides past without touching me, doesn't carry me away or hold me in its grip.

I now play second violin, third actually, and even that I still have to learn.

A short pause with a cup of tea outside in the cool mountain air allows me to take out my earplugs for a while.

After a muffled second part, where my earplugs also serve me well against the prolonged enthusiastic applause, we walk down the mountain at an easy pace.

Am I really getting better? In any case, things are definitely different.

Back in the Netherlands, Willem again asks me to go to the opera. I can sleep on it for a night before deciding. This is also the first time I can do this: go to sleep with a decision waiting to be taken. But is it really necessary? Before going to sleep I already know the opera is a bad idea. If I say yes I will be unapproachable for the whole weekend and nobody will understand why. On the contrary, they will cheerfully suggest yet another activity for Saturday and preferably yet another for Sunday.

I wish they would leave me in peace. I no longer want my life to be ruled by the fact that I can't use my brain for long periods of time and that my body won't listen to me. I don't want to be dominated by pain, I want to rein in the pain and lead it into manageable paths.

Does this mean that all my longings for music are extinguished? No, certainly not. But I have to ignore or suppress them. In any case I don't want to fall into self-pity. And I must not let myself be coerced into going along.

'You'll be sitting peacefully all evening, won't you?'

Yes, maybe so, but my senses will be wide-open and the cacophony of sounds from the orchestra will torment my ears. To some extent I can close down my senses. I have some experience with this by now. Earplugs in, dark glasses on! Don't look at people or follow them with your eyes. Don't start conversations, don't chat during the interval. And stay in your seat, since walking is impossible.

But even when I eliminate all these stimuli, I won't be able to sleep for nights! Why am I even considering it? It's sheer madness to go to the opera.

Be smart, Andrea, you can't do anything about it. Stay home and enjoy your umpteenth 'free' evening. Stay home alone, take rest, and go to bed in time.

The next morning I advise Willem about whom he could invite to Bizet's *Carmen*.

And now Willem is dissatisfied with my performance as hostess. As he sees it, I don't do a thing about it. Not a soul comes to dinner anymore. Our house is dead as a doornail. Never anything happening. And that is just one aspect of a task I had always carried out with great pleasure and energy.

I stop up my ears. 'I don't want to hear about it!' To defend myself I shout that I am a poor excuse for the woman I used to be. A washed-out little wimp. Yeah, yeah,

I know, he misses me as his little golf buddy, always up for a game, and he hates having to turn down all those invitations, or going to dinner parties where I am conspicuous by my absence, or showing up at receptions without me by his side, always having to explain to his colleagues and clients and the employees and co-directors from his office that I am still a long way from recovery.

It's true, we no longer invite large groups of people to our home. Giving birthday parties, let alone organizing them, has become an impossible task for me. We don't go out in the evenings anymore, not to the movies, or to restaurants, or to theaters or concerts.

And now Willem is fed up with it. He thinks we don't have a life anymore. Good grief, Willem is really starting to get sick of it all.

So on top of everything else this lands on my plate. I try to talk him round a little but that takes so much effort I go to the bedroom, totally exhausted, with an aching brain and a face on fire.

But I know from experience that I must deal with his complaints without delay. Otherwise he will cloak himself in a stubborn silence and that's the last thing I want. This fire of discontent must be extinguished straightaway, even if I feel totally rotten afterwards. I'm not going to let myself be robbed of both my health and my husband by some snot-nosed punk on a moped.

I start out bravely: 'If you want to bellyache, don't put it on me but on that hoodlum who caused all this. If you're a real man, do something about dealing with these traffic criminals, but don't chew out your brain-injured wife. I've been through enough. And I'm already stretched to my limit! Do you have any idea how many times I have to stop myself thinking about things I want to do? Do you ever consider that? I wobble around like an idiot and have to ignore all my skills and talents. And to make matters worse you saddle me with a guilty conscience by scolding me for not functioning properly. As if I didn't know that already!'

The tears well up, but I don't want to cry.

I go on: 'There are only a very few people who have really been important for us in this time of heavy trials. Wonderful people, who were always there for us and supported us. They listened to all those strange and unfamiliar complaints that go with contusio cerebri. They had never heard anything about it before, but they listened to our stories, time and time again. They helped us, each in their own way, said the right thing at the right time, an art that few people seem to understand, helped us think things through and thought up situations in which I could be happy, thought about how I could keep my balance better, how I could protect my injured neck and my oversensitive ears and eyes.

These are the only people for whom I would like to organize anything. Inviting them all at once is no longer possible and we'll need to choose a good time, so I won't have to be punished for it with sleepless nights. A brunch in the weekend, around noon, would be best for me. And I will really have to push myself to the limit to pull it off.'

So we give four brunches, each time with two guests who stay two or three hours. Afterwards I'm totally bushed and zigzag off to bed. Rest and peace, windows open. Sons wanting to talk to me are told to go away. And then a restless night.

But what else am I supposed to do? How else am I supposed to satisfy my need to communicate with good people?

If they asked me sincerely, I would rather see no one, but no one asks me sincerely and I would not answer sincerely anyway.

Who is suffering anything as unfathomable as this affliction of mine?

The Great Silence

At nine o'clock on a Sunday morning I am wakened by a throbbing wave of noise. There seems to be no end to it. The first thing that pops into my head is that an airplane is making an emergency landing in our garden.

Willem and I pull on our bathrobes and hurry outside. We see a long unbroken column of motorcyclists riding three abreast at high speed down our street, taking up the whole road. We feel powerless in the face of such a mass of noise and stench and make no attempt to disguise our indignation. I wrench myself out of Willem's protective grasp and stand in the middle of the road as a living blockade to make the motorcyclists reduce their speed and ride one behind the other.

My action has some effect, but imagine my amazement when I see a police car accompanying the column.

Once back inside, our whole kitchen reeks of exhaust fumes.

What I love best is to be in an environment where the harshest disturbers of the peace are the crickets in the grass, the buzzing insects, the leaves rustling in the wind, and the cowbells. The German names of the houses in the village where we like to stay reflect the peace of the surroundings: *Abendruh, Almenrausch, Alpenruh, Bergruh...*

The house rules of our village apartment are also clear on the subject: 'In the interest of harmonious relations with their neighbors, all tenants are obliged to ensure that there is no noise pollution caused, for example, by radios, loud conversation, slamming doors, etc. Between 10 p.m.

147

and 8 a.m., tenants must take care to do nothing that would disturb their neighbors' rest. Walking in hiking boots and moving furniture back and forth is to be avoided. It is strictly forbidden to wear ski boots in the house.'

In early 1900, Winston Churchill spent some time in a villa just above our village. While he was there, his study and writing were so disturbed by the penetrating clang of cowbells that it began to get seriously on his nerves. He thought it over carefully and decided to strike a compromise with the cowherds, paying them to stuff the bells with hay and grass.

A number of years ago the same thing happened to us. Just below our house grazed a herd of huge cows with equally huge bells. No problem in the daytime, but at night we couldn't sleep a wink. We put our problem to the director of the local tourist bureau and the herd was moved to a meadow higher up the mountain.

People with brain injuries are extra-sensitive to noise. Unfortunately, no one seems to take this into consideration. Or almost no one. On a cold but sunny Fall day three years after my accident, in the nature sanctuary near my little writing retreat, the racket caused by two low-flying pleasure planes and a helicopter nearly drove me out of my mind.

In a rare moment of silence I heard the geese preparing for their winter migration. Since I couldn't hear very well in this sanctuary full of droning aircraft, I was happy with the visual confirmation provided by their V-formation.

Then one of the pleasure craft really went too far, buzzing the fields at a threateningly low altitude. The sheep won't protest, the pilot must have thought. But I was there too. With my crimson jacket on, I reckoned the clown could see me clearly. I stood still and elaborately covered my ears with my hands. To my surprise, he stopped circling so near to the ground. His zooming and roaring faded away into a distant monotonous drone.

I could hear the cackling of the geese again. When I walked back to the house I could even hear the sound of the grazing sheep.

Despite the fact that the Netherlands has something like a thousand federal environment officials, there seems to be very little policy on air and noise pollution.

Apparently, the air is still free. Even the Civil Aviation Authority has nothing to say about it.

In this connection, sociologist Prof. A.C. Zijderveld speaks of auditory environmental pollution, auditory torment and physical pain in the auditory channels. In a newspaper article entitled 'Silence and noise' he writes: 'Silence has become the scarcest commodity is our prosperous society. Only in remote natural areas, high in the mountains or on the tundra or in distant forests, can we still experience silence as an almost physical, corporeal reality.' He goes on: 'Apparently, construction workers have acquired the right to auditory environmental pollution as part of the fringe benefits under their collective bargaining agreements. Academic white-collar workers have no agreements guaranteeing their right to silence.'

The lampposts on our street are getting their yearly overhaul. A truck with its motor running is parked in front of our house. Two young men are sitting in the cabin with earsplitting pop music pouring out of the open windows. I walk up with my hands over my ears. With evident reluctance, they turn down the radio so that they can understand me. 'Is there a problem?'

'Yes, there is! Why does it sound like a house party is going on in my home when the music is coming out of your radio?'

'We're working here!'

'Fine, but would you please put on headphones? Then you have your music but I don't have to listen to it.'

Loud protest. Until I play my last, authoritative trump: 'Do I have to call your boss?'

Luckily the gentlemen decide not to test me further.

A national newspaper announces the foundation of a Dutch association to combat acoustic pollution. Apparently, hundreds of letters testify that people are thrown into a chaotic state by the muzak they are subjected to while shopping. They come home with the wrong things or forget to buy the things they need because they are unable to concentrate properly.

In the same article professor of experimental psychology Piet Vroon states that unasked-for noise lowers people's level of activity. It is difficult to carry out complicated tasks under such circumstances.

Patients with brain and whiplash injuries could be an important target group for the new association, since the best remedy for all these patients is peace and quiet.

'I step aside for no one, except the horse and cart' we used to sing as children when we proclaimed the street our playground and defended our newly won territory by playing on obliviously in defiance of the traffic, only jumping to the safety of the sidewalk at the very last

150

moment. The only exception we made was for the horses of the men who went about collecting waste and old clothes in their carts, that we could pet and feed old bread.

When cars took over the streets, the petting stopped.

My Co-victim

Do I sometimes sit and cry all on my own? No, unfortunately not. I do it especially for my husband. You could set your watch by it. When he comes home in the evening and asks on his way to his study, 'How did it go today?', I am sure to burst into an unstoppable flood of tears. Then he comes back and sits down with a pile of letters and faxes at the dinner table. Lots of rustling and crackling, noises I simply can't stand. And the tears keep flowing.

'Hey, you're crying? Does the noise bother you? I'll be gone in a minute.'

With his arm around my shoulder Willem listens to my lamentations, eats quickly, gives me a kiss and leaves again. 'I'm concerned about you', he tells me, 'but I can't do anything to help. See you later!'

'But by then I'll be in bed already.'

Through the car window I hear him say, 'Well, there's nothing I can do about that,'

I see him off with a lump in my throat. There's nothing to blame him for. It's not his job to look after my bruised brain.

I can't do much to change this situation. How am I supposed to keep the daily crying jags within bounds? Am I sometimes just whining for attention?

My life in the twilight zone is no longer bearable. It just goes on and on and on. One day after another, like endless beads on a string. Days filled with an aching head, so that the most normal things in the world become unattainable.

Am I progressing? Regressing? Who keeps me in touch, who gives me heart in this impossible struggle? Does anyone understand what I'm going through? That my head is good for almost nothing and can be used for just minutes each day? That I have trouble standing erect like a human being?

Often, my greatest longing is to go lie down in a room by myself, but I have to repress it. I am literally pulling myself through the days. Brain cells take an agonizingly long time to recover.

No, I don't cry to get attention. Willem's working habits haven't changed at all, so that's not the problem.

In fact I maneuver myself into this impossible position. A normal person with this pain and deathly fatigue would simply stay in bed, but I have set myself the task of serving my husband and children a homemade hot meal every day, just as I did before the accident. Is that aiming too high?

The kitchen where I am busy all afternoon, preparing a salad at my own slow pace, is transformed into a dim grayish mass, and the presence of another person only makes my floundering and fumbling worse.

Willem has already gotten used to taking our hot meal out of the microwave himself, so that he needn't be confronted with the sight of my hopeless wobbly shuffle past the sink.

But that doesn't solve my problems. I can no longer sit up properly. I am exhausted. Certainly in no condition to listen to people's stories, not even those of my darling Willem. I push myself through this hardest part of the day, hoping only to go soon to the seclusion of my bed.

To go to bed and sleep might well be a solution, but it is not that simple. I am obviously incapable of running my house like clockwork. And if we don't sit down to dinner together I will never see my husband at all. By the time I finally dress myself at ten or eleven in the morning he is long gone. And when he comes home at night he finds me totally unapproachable in bed again.

This may be the best way to fulfil my great longing for peace and quiet, but even a good marriage could fall to pieces under such a well-nigh unbearable burden.

So, out of necessity, I take a hard road, even though it weighs heavily on both of us. One important reason for keeping up my cooking duties is the boost I get from mastering this domestic task again to some extent. Thus I spend hours on my own doing what I consider to be useful work.

The second reason is that communication always makes inroads on my energy, and I try to conserve my verbal energy as much as possible for Willem, who is entitled to it more than anyone. I would do anything to preserve our relationship.

If I lost him too, I would be even worse off!

'It must be no fun for your husband either!' was a remark that still made me furious even two years after the accident. My caustic retort was always the same: 'I'd be happy to trade with him!'.

Amazed look.

Which really got me going: 'He had to miss four whole days of work! I'm still a zombie, incapable of functioning normally. There's just no comparison.'

You could forget about any sympathy from me. Only four years after the accident was I somewhat capable of empathy: 'Yes, it must have been quite a shock!'

Willem still tells other people: 'My wife is a patient.' Unnoticed by me, people will no doubt agree with him. But due to the great reduction in human contacts, I never hear the word 'patient'. That isn't necessarily a drawback, as I thought at first. No, there are things you would rather not hear.

It is mainly on vacation that he has to face the facts.

God, he made me mad the first time he came up with that remark. I was outraged and dumbfounded. When he kept hammering away at it, I could have strangled him. 'Do you want to trade?' I needled him. 'See who gets depressive first with contusio cerebri?'

Now that there are so few things we can do together, I can well imagine how 'lonely' he must feel. He has to go everywhere on his own, while we used to do everything, or almost everything, together. He looks like a divorced man.

I console him by telling him he should make the most of being able to go everywhere and meet and talk to people. I would love to come along. And didn't I often go alone to PTA meetings and birthdays in the past? And did I make such a fuss about it?

I know that this comparison doesn't really apply, but what else am I supposed to say to cheer him up?

Willem is what is known as a co-victim. But how far are we to stretch this concept? The circle of co-victims keeps getting bigger, widening to include relatives, housemates and even nurses and perpetrators. Where does this kind of thinking end? And why do co-victims only pop

155

up in cases of sickness, death and misery? Don't birth and divorce create co-victims too?

Now and then we go off for a few days to the sand dunes of North Holland, the lakes of Friesland or the woodlands near the German border. It's enough to make me very happy. I have to fight hard to get away, for my once so quick-witted speech now generally deteriorates into stutter and stammer.

I slowly realize that I have to come up with alternatives myself if I want us to do something together, no matter how much energy it costs me. If I hand over the reins our outings turn into fiascoes.

We have booked spacious accommodation in a nice hotel in the eastern Netherlands. It turns out to be a suite with a cozy little kitchenette, so we don't have go to the restaurant every time we want a cup of coffee. The only things missing are a writing table and two chairs, but the owner's son soon brings them, along with some extra wood for the open fireplace.

We explore the surroundings on hotel bikes: no freeway noises, only tractors, sheep and the smell of pigs. We stop in a little village to buy wine, a corkscrew, soup and tea, and with the box under the carrier straps we ride back home.

After dinner Willem watches television for awhile and I leaf through my magazines. At ten-thirty it's nearly past my bedtime. Just when Willem decides to do a little work on his computer.

And here we go again. I am sleeping in an office.

I manage to refrain from explaining everything to him again in minute detail, realizing that the main thing is not to add to my problems by getting all worked up about it.

But how can Willem be so inconsiderate as to start tapping and bleeping away on his computer in our bedroom at ten-thirty at night? Can't he see that I want to sleep and am already troubled by an easily irritated head?

No, he really can't stop, he says, a couple of things just have to be finished.

That's it, never again. How can I avoid such situations in the future? At home the risk of irritation has been removed because Willem and his computer stay in his own territory, but not here.

In the house in the mountains he went out on the balcony to sit and work and make noises with his new laptop, preferably with the telephone next to him. After all, that's what all this portable equipment is for, to work and make a racket wherever you are.

But I managed to put a stop to that. Silence on the balcony, silence in the living room, silence in the bedroom. He can bleep and telephone to his heart's delight in his splendid study, with the door closed.

The burden is almost too much for my head. The price is high, and is this how I want to spend my very precious time here?

I have no choice. I have more need than ever for solitude and my own space. Otherwise I will no longer be able to live with him.

In May we stayed in Andalusia. The apartment was spacious, light and pleasant, with all modern conveniences. Two bathrooms and two bedrooms offered interesting possibilities. Willem had transformed the living-cum-dining room into an office, where he phoned, faxed and modemed, so that his work went on as usual. Publications were launched and books finalized. I sat at the marble table on the balcony. Apart yet together. This disciplined arrangement was very much to my liking. It was almost like home.

A little swimming pool and a tennis court were located on the roof. You took the elevator to the fourth floor, then up a steep stairway without banister to the fifth, where the last step was too narrow to allow you to open the door while standing on it. So I had to take a step backwards, a step down, in other words, with my swimming gear in my arms. Under these difficult conditions, I managed to maintain my shaky balance only with the greatest possible care. The razor-sharp marble steps and rough stucco walls made the idea of tumbling downstairs exceptionally unattractive.

Finally I had a bedroom of my own. What luxury, finally no need for my arms to hang out of bed half the night. When I sat up I could not only smell but see the sea. Through the sliding door I could step right out onto the balcony, with its view of the Rock of Gibraltar.

There was a complete bathroom attached. I went to bed at ten and got up again at nine. I would wake at six, but thanks to the roll-down shutters and insulating curtains go peacefully back to sleep. With Willem next to me I wouldn't sleep a wink.

Since the accident I found my husband and bedmate much harder to bear. His nocturnal habits were very irritating, even agitating to me. But nobody disturbed my sleep here.

Willem complains about loss of intimacy. It seems to make him happy just to lie next to that inert body of mine and disturb my rest.

His need for intimacy is different than mine. His intimacy is oppressive to me. But can I compare myself to people without contusio cerebri? I actually have more need for support to be able to go on living in this totally rotten way.

My need for Willem is much greater than it used to be, but not at all when I am sleeping, not in my immediate vicinity where I can so easily be disturbed by noise. I must protect myself, for I don't think I am completely normal.

'Don't disturb me and leave me alone when I ask you to.'

And all that drivel about intimacy when you're asleep!

I don't sleep well next to someone who's sneezing and tossing and turning and who goes to bed much later than I do and gets up much earlier.

My medicine is 'leave me in peace'.

During one of many sleepless nights I write Willem a letter, weeping over my hopeless situation. For days now, he has cloaked himself stubbornly in stoic silence. It is driving me mad. How can I reach him with my limited energy?

I must cut through a Gordian knot. I may have injured my brain, but I won't let my soul be harmed. That's where I draw the line.

I write:

Willem,

Too bad I wasn't killed outright. I wouldn't have been a burden to you then. A death is soon forgotten. Life goes on. In time you would have found another woman to make you happy! And that's something I wouldn't grudge you.

I didn't dare utter this death wish earlier, for then a whole little army of psychologists would have crawled all over me, saying 'Madam is depressed', sticking that kind of label on me.

But things turned out otherwise. I didn't die, didn't lose my IQ, just my social life. That has been reduced to zero. And the social life we shared together, with all its varied aspects, has suffered the same fate. Nonetheless I feel fairly stable again, supported more by structures I've devised myself than by other people.

When you keep looking straight through me the few times I see you I really die inside. That silent treatment is deadly.

I realize that you miss my presence in various situations, but in this we share the same fate. Funny, isn't it? No, you don't find anything funny right now.

Your reactions are characterized by angry and sullen behavior. You are so remote that conversation is practically impossible. While I avoid other conversations and activities so that I can be in the best state possible for our weekends together, usually without the children. So when you suddenly surprise me with the news that you are not going to be there this evening, I get furious. You look defiant, but mainly indifferent. Not a word crosses your lips. I dig in my heels, and make my plan.

That I hereby submit to you:

If you can't find the time in your busy weekend schedule to do something with me, no matter how little, that's not my problem. I can't do the impossible.

There's no sense in talking, you say, since that can't change my situation. But then you had better just put an end to your marriage right now. A dead end. Then I can make other arrangements to carry on with my (limited) life. A life in which I will stand up for myself very selfishly. Now I'm just trailing along after you like a spineless idiot. I'll still be an idiot of course. But what I will gain is the time I now spend on you. That time will then be my own.

For God's sake don't stay with me out of pity or duty or because it's the proper thing to do. Only stay because you love me, with all my limitations. You have a few of your own, you know!

This past weekend I needed a crowbar to get through to you. It may sound interesting to deal with a husband as silent as the tomb, but nothing could be further from the truth. Nor is it the first time you fall silent, but under the present circumstances I am no longer able to solve your communication problems for you. I'm completely fed up with it. I'm on strike.

My weekly schedule consists entirely of managing our household. I order all our provisions and other purchases by fax and look after everything that needs to be done in this respect. When the old house needs repairs you point to me and say that I can

161

handle it. You can throw yourself completely into your work. 'Cleaning' is not part of your vocabulary, but 'delegating' is. That's the way it was and that's the way it still is after my contusio cerebri.

The fact that I would like to vanish from your life is the crowbar I'm using to break open your mouth after days of silence. And you know I mean it, I will not allow myself to be deliberately wounded. Luckily, I am still able to protect my heart. I know for sure that it is in the right place.

I am totally dumbfounded to hear that you feel depressed lately due to my hopeless situation. Nothing can be changed about it and you are sabotaged in everything you want to do because of my limitations. While before... It drives me completely wild! I have the handicap and he gets depressed! No way I can look on the bright side here. I thought sufficient alternatives had been developed by now to meet certain needs. Wrong again. Even then he still gets depressed. Just like he used to, by the way, but since I came into his life the skies have nearly always been sunny.

Not so long ago you were enthusiastically reading out to me passages from Winslade's *Confronting Traumatic Brain Injury*. As a co-victim, you told me, you could easily identify with the five stages experienced by someone going through a mourning process. You find that what Kuebler-Ross calls the stages of shock and denial, anger, depression, bargaining and finally acceptance are applicable to my situation. Yet, you said, the partner's mourning process takes a quite different course with brain injury than it does with death. You told me you keep being confronted with two things Kuebler-Ross doesn't mention. On the one hand with my changeable and uncertain recovery process, on the other with the necessity of facing the trauma day after day, again and again, making it impossible for you to distance yourself from it. You told me it is practically inevitable for the partner of someone suffering from brain injury to fall into depression.

You are also troubled by guilt feelings, you confess. That doesn't shock me, and you can do something about it by changing your behavior. If you think I get too little attention, you can leave a blank spot for my name in your schedule each week. If you would rather fill in someone else's name, I'd like to know about it, so that I can make my own choices. But you can only create space in your weekend schedule by cutting back either on your work or your golf.

The choice is up to you. If you say it's certainly worth doing for me, and I look skeptical as usual, well, that's your problem.

For the time being, what it implies for me is simply to wait and see how you solve this problem in practice.

Epilogue

He looks at me with his friendly, scrutinizing eyes. He wants an answer. Preferably a positive answer that I am alright, that I'm all better! Did I do anything fun during his five-day absence when he was at a conference abroad? He notices that I want to laugh. Yes, I actually did do fun things: a former member of my student society came to visit, we had coffee in the sun and talked, trying to bridge almost forty years, which was nearly impossible in that one short hour; I rode my bicycle to deliver a belated birthday present to my godson; I surprised a neighbour with blooming hydrangea branches and sat with her in her garden for a short while; I bought a sunny bathing suit. No, I didn't go to the swimming pool yet: I haven't had the time. Now my husband starts to laugh "I hope you didn't try to cram all these activities into one day?' Instead of shrugging it off I become defensive: 'No, of course not, I've learned my lesson and only do one activity a day and with a rest day in between. You know those visits drain my energy, so after the news it's off to bed, exhausted.'
'Yes, well', he grumbles, 'tell me something I haven't heard before …'

Still, I feel good about the past few days. What I do may not seem very exciting to an outsider, but I am more than happy with it. I am actually like the mice that play when the cat's away. Minus the playing, that is. But I am glad he is home again, because without him my life would not run as smoothly as it does now. My husband can do at least three activities in one day and I - on the best of days - can do one. He is also the one who, quick as lightning, my calendar in his hand, makes a series of appointments for some medical check-ups, telephones the GP to have him prepare the necessary referral letters so I can collect them that afternoon on my bike. If that isn't love.

And when I am happily riding my bicycle I often hear the question: 'Wow, you're getting better all the time, aren't you?' And I nod affirmatively. But I don't tell them that going out or meeting friends until the wee hours of the morning is no longer an option. That my gear is always in reverse. That going a hundred miles an hour is out of the question for me, because I'd be wiped out after ten minutes. That I have considerably less 'fit hours' than many other people. Today my husband and I live our own, highly soloistic lives. He gets al lot done in little time and I get little done in a lot of time. After watching the news, for example, he will do some work whereas I am in my bed again! Apparently we have adjusted our behaviour enough to be able to cope with this often very oppressive and restrictive situation. But countless are the times we have managed to avoid immanent derailment so far. It has proven to be a tall order.

So has nothing good come from this accident? Well, that is one of those questions! What am I supposed to answer? I would still rather be an active octopus than a slow tortoise. I prefer to emphasize the sunny side of the story. The book, the Contusio Cerebri Fund Foundation with its website www.hersenkneuzing.nl and the many hours spent on it by the editors are positive developments after such a disastrous event. It brings new meaning to my quiet and withdrawn life. It makes this life, with all its limitations, worth living for me and also for others who have suffered the same fate. I hope the website helps make the information about concussion and contusion of the brain accessible for other victims and their families, but also for all care professionals.

———